Title: LOW GLYCEMIC MEALS

Balancing Blood Sugar with Delicious and Healthy Recipes

By

Nancy Bratton

First published by Nancy Bratton 2024
Copyright © 2024 by Nancy Bratton

Introduction   **5**

Demystifying the Glycemic Index: Your Key to Balanced Blood Sugar and Steady Energy   6

The Importance of Incorporating Low Glycemic Meals   7

Real-Life Stories of Health Transformation with Low Glycemic Eating   10

Chapter 1: Understanding the Glycemic Index   **15**

Factors Influencing Glycemic Index   17

Benefits of Low Glycemic Foods   18

Foods to eat on the low glycemic diet   22

Foods to avoid on the low glycemic diet   25

Chapter 2: Identifying Low Glycemic Foods   **29**

Characteristics of Low Glycemic Foods   32

Practical Tips for Incorporating Low Glycemic Foods   35

Chapter 3: Healthy and Nutritious Low Glycemic Breakfast Recipes   **41**

Chapter 4: Nutrient-Dense Low Glycemic Lunch Recipes   **79**

Chapter 5: Healthy and Nutritious Low Glycemic Dinner Feast Recipes   **151**

Chapter 6:Nutrient-Dense Low Glycemic Desserts and Snacks   **201**

   50 nutrient-dense low glycemic snack recipes: 235

Chapter 7:Low Glycemic Nutrient-dense Meal Plan 257

Conclusion   **289**

Daily Meal Remark   **291**

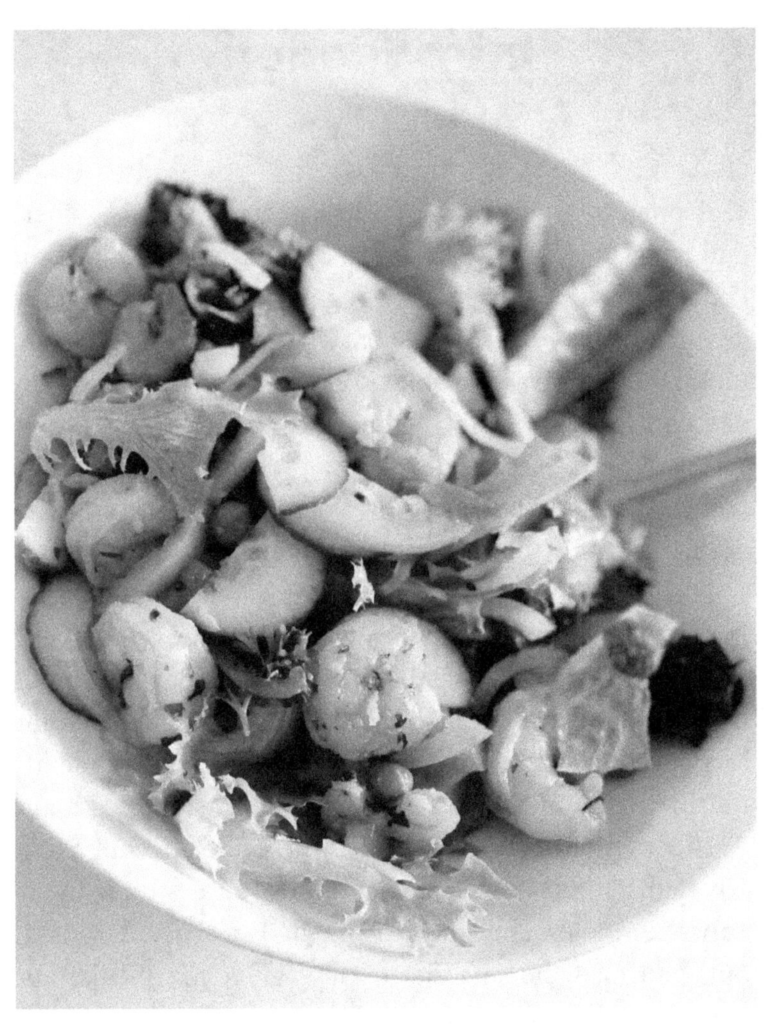

Introduction

Welcome to the world of low glycemic meals, where delicious meets healthy! In this book, we'll explore the concept of low glycemic eating, its benefits for overall health, and how to create satisfying meals that keep your blood sugar levels stable. Whether you're managing diabetes, trying to lose weight, or simply seeking to improve your eating habits, low glycemic meals offer a wealth of benefits. Get ready to embark on a journey of culinary delight and nutritional excellence!

In today's fast-paced world, where processed foods and sugary snacks are readily available, maintaining a healthy diet can be challenging. However, understanding and incorporating low glycemic meals into your daily routine can significantly improve your overall health and well-being. However, we will explore the concept of the Glycemic Index (GI), we can unlock a treasure trove of delicious meals that nourish our bodies from the inside out, and also the benefits of low glycemic meals, and why they are essential for long-term health.

Demystifying the Glycemic Index: Your Key to Balanced Blood Sugar and Steady Energy

Have you ever noticed a mid-afternoon slump hit you like a ton of bricks? Or maybe you experience ravenous hunger pangs shortly after a seemingly satisfying meal? These energy crashes and cravings can often be attributed to the way your body processes carbohydrates and how they impact your blood sugar levels. Enter the Glycemic Index (GI), a powerful tool for understanding how different foods affect your energy and overall well-being.

Think of the GI as a rating system, like one you might use for movies. Instead of emotions evoked on screen, the GI ranks carbohydrate-containing foods on a scale of 0 to 100 based on their impact on blood sugar (glucose) levels. Here's the key: the higher the GI score, the faster your blood sugar rises after consuming that food. Conversely, low GI foods cause a gradual and sustained increase in blood sugar.

Let's break it down further:

The Reference Point (GI 100): Imagine pure glucose, the simplest form of sugar, as our reference point. It gets absorbed into the bloodstream rapidly, spiking blood sugar levels quickly. Hence, it has a GI of 100.

The Slow and Steady Climbers (Low GI): These champions, like lentils, sweet potatoes, and whole grains, are digested and absorbed at a slower pace. This translates to a gentle rise in blood sugar, keeping you energized and your mind sharp for longer.

The Sugar Rockets (High GI): These are the culprits behind those energy crashes. Think white bread, sugary breakfast cereals, and processed snacks. They cause a rapid surge in blood sugar, followed by an inevitable crash as your body releases insulin to manage the spike. This rollercoaster ride can leave you feeling drained and yearning for another sugary fix.

Understanding the GI of foods is crucial for making informed dietary choices, especially for individuals with diabetes, those looking to manage their weight, or anyone interested in maintaining stable energy levels throughout the day.

The Importance of Incorporating Low Glycemic Meals

Incorporating low glycemic meals into your diet is not just about managing blood sugar levels or losing weight; it's about fostering a sustainable, healthy lifestyle. By focusing on foods that promote gradual glucose release, you can enjoy consistent energy levels, reduce the risk of chronic diseases, and enhance your quality of life.

Transitioning to a low glycemic diet may require some initial adjustments, such as becoming familiar with the GI values of different foods and planning balanced meals. However, the long-term benefits far outweigh the effort, leading to a healthier, more vibrant life.

Understanding and embracing the concept of low glycemic meals is a powerful step towards better health. Whether you are looking to manage a medical condition, achieve weight loss goals, or simply enhance your overall well-being, a diet rich in low glycemic foods offers numerous advantages. This guide will provide you with the knowledge and tools needed to make informed choices, helping you to incorporate low glycemic meals into your everyday life for sustained health benefits.

Now that you have a solid understanding of the GI, you're well on your way to making informed choices about the carbohydrates you consume. Let's explore a delicious world of low GI meals that will keep you energized, satisfied, and thriving!

In this book, we'll dive deep into the world of low glycemic eating, exploring the science behind it, its myriad benefits, and practical strategies for incorporating it into your lifestyle. From breakfast to dessert, we'll provide you with a treasure trove of delicious recipes and meal ideas that prove healthy eating doesn't have to be boring or restrictive.

So, whether you're a seasoned health enthusiast or just starting your journey towards better nutrition, get ready to embark on a culinary adventure that will tantalize your taste buds, nourish your body, and leave you feeling energized and empowered. Welcome to the world of low glycemic meals – where delicious meets healthy, and every bite brings you one step closer to vibrant well-being.

Real-Life Stories of Health Transformation with Low Glycemic Eating

John's Journey to Steady Energy Levels

John, a 45-year-old accountant, was constantly battling energy crashes throughout his workday. "I used to rely on coffee and sugary snacks to get through the afternoon slump," John recalls. "It felt like a never-ending cycle of highs and lows." Frustrated with his fluctuating energy levels and weight gain, John decided to make a change. He started following a low glycemic diet after reading about its benefits.

"Switching to low glycemic meals was a game-changer," John says. ""I started my mornings with hearty breakfasts like overnight chia pudding, which kept me satisfied and energized until lunchtime." The crashes disappeared, and I was more productive at work." Within a few months, John not only stabilized his energy levels but also shed 15 pounds. "I feel like a new person. This lifestyle has truly transformed my health."

Emily's Path to Better Blood Sugar Control

Emily, a 32-year-old teacher, was diagnosed with prediabetes. Concerned about her future health, she sought ways to manage her blood sugar levels naturally. "I was scared when I got my diagnosis," Emily shares. "I knew I had to make a change, but I didn't want to rely solely on medication."

Emily discovered the benefits of low glycemic eating and decided to give it a try. "I started incorporating more low glycemic foods into my diet—lots of vegetables, whole grains, and lean proteins," she explains. "I was pleasantly surprised by how tasty and fulfilling the meals turned out to be.

Over time, Emily's blood sugar levels improved significantly. "My doctor was amazed at my progress. My A1C levels dropped to a healthy range, and I felt more in control of my health." Emily's story is a testament to the power of dietary changes in managing blood sugar levels naturally.

Mark and Sarah's Family Transformation

Mark and Sarah, parents to two young children, were struggling to maintain a healthy lifestyle amidst their busy schedules. "We were always grabbing fast food or quick, processed meals," Sarah admits. "We knew we needed to set a better example for our kids."

The couple decided to embark on a low glycemic eating journey together. "We started meal planning and cooking together," Mark says. "It turned into a fun family activity, and we all eagerly anticipated experimenting with new recipes together".

The results were astounding. "We all felt more energetic and focused," Sarah notes. "The kids even enjoyed the new meals, and we saw improvements in their behavior and concentration." Mark and Sarah also noticed weight loss and better overall health. "It brought us closer as a family and transformed our approach to food."

Linda's Weight Loss Success

Linda, a 50-year-old marketing executive, had struggled with weight management for years. "I tried every diet out there, but nothing seemed to work long-term," Linda says. "I was always hungry and frustrated."

A friend recommended a low glycemic diet, and Linda decided to give it a try. "I was skeptical at first, but I was desperate for a solution," she recalls. "I began by making simple changes, such as replacing high-glycemic foods with healthier options."

To her surprise, Linda found the diet easy to follow and incredibly satisfying. ""I didn't feel hungry constantly, and I didn't have to obsessively count calories," she explains. Over the course of a year, Linda lost 30 pounds and kept it off. "It's been life-changing. I have more energy, my mood has improved, and I feel confident again."

Paul's Improved Heart Health

Paul, a 60-year-old retiree, was diagnosed with high cholesterol and hypertension. "I knew I needed to make serious changes to my diet," Paul says. "My doctor suggested a low glycemic diet to help manage my cholesterol and blood pressure."

Paul embraced the new eating plan with determination. "I started incorporating more fiber-rich foods, healthy fats, and lean proteins into my meals," he explains. "It was a big shift, but the recipes in 'Low Glycemic Meals' made it easier."

Within six months, Paul's cholesterol levels improved significantly, and his blood pressure normalized. "My doctor was impressed with my progress," Paul shares. "I feel healthier and more active than I have in years.

Embracing a low glycemic diet was the best decision I made for my heart health."

These and many more are real-life stories that highlight the transformative power of low glycemic eating. Whether it's stabilizing energy levels, managing blood sugar, improving family health, achieving weight loss, or enhancing heart health, adopting a low glycemic diet can lead to remarkable improvements in overall well-being. These individuals' experiences serve as inspiring examples of how making mindful dietary choices can have a profound impact on one's health and quality of life.

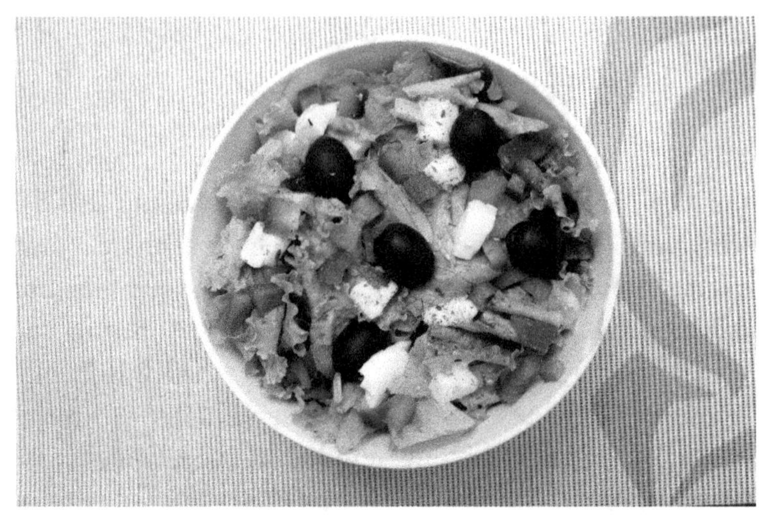

Chapter 1: Understanding the Glycemic Index

The Glycemic Index (GI) is a vital tool for anyone looking to improve their dietary habits and overall health. By understanding how different foods affect blood glucose levels, you can make more informed decisions that support long-term wellness. This chapter delves into the fundamentals of the Glycemic Index, its development, and its practical applications in everyday life.

The Concept of the Glycemic Index

What is the Glycemic Index?

The Glycemic Index is a numerical system that rates carbohydrates based on how quickly they are converted into glucose and absorbed into the bloodstream. Developed in the early 1980s by Dr. David Jenkins and colleagues at the University of Toronto, the GI helps to categorize foods into three main groups:

- Low GI Foods (0-55): These foods produce a slow, steady increase in blood sugar levels.
- Medium GI Foods (56-69): These foods result in a moderate rise in blood sugar levels.
- High GI Foods (70-100): These foods cause a rapid spike in blood sugar levels.

How the Glycemic Index is Measured

The GI of a food is determined through clinical testing. Typically, 10 or more healthy participants consume a portion of the test food containing 50 grams of available carbohydrates. Their blood glucose levels are then measured at regular intervals over a two-hour period. This data is compared to the response elicited by a reference food, usually glucose or white bread, which is assigned a GI value of 100. The resulting blood glucose response of the test food is expressed as a percentage of the reference food, providing its GI value.

Factors Influencing Glycemic Index

Several factors can affect the GI of a food, including:

- **Type of Carbohydrate:** Simple sugars tend to have a higher GI compared to complex carbohydrates.
- **Fiber Content:** Foods high in soluble fiber typically have a lower GI because fiber slows down digestion.
- **Fat and Protein Content:** The presence of fat and protein can lower the GI of a food by slowing gastric emptying.
- **Food Processing:** Processed foods generally have a higher GI than their whole, unprocessed counterparts.
- **Ripeness**: For fruits and vegetables, the level of ripeness can affect their GI; riper fruits have higher GI values.
- **Cooking Method:** How a food is cooked can also influence its GI. For example, al dente pasta has a lower GI than soft-cooked pasta.

Benefits of Low Glycemic Foods

Understanding the benefits of low glycemic foods can help you appreciate why integrating them into your diet is advantageous.

The benefits of low glycemic eating extend far beyond blood sugar control. Research has shown that adopting a low GI diet can aid in weight management by reducing cravings and promoting feelings of fullness. It can also improve insulin sensitivity, lower the risk of heart disease, and even enhance cognitive function.

Whether you're managing diabetes, trying to shed a few pounds, or simply striving to optimize your health, incorporating low glycemic meals into your diet can be a game-changer. And the best part? You don't have to sacrifice taste or variety. With a little creativity and know-how, you can enjoy a wide array of mouthwatering dishes that satisfy your cravings while nourishing your body.

1. Improved Blood Sugar Control

One of the primary benefits of consuming low glycemic meals is the stabilization of blood sugar levels. Unlike high GI foods, which cause rapid spikes and subsequent crashes in blood sugar, low GI foods provide a more controlled release of glucose into the bloodstream. This helps prevent the energy dips and cravings often associated with fluctuating blood sugar levels.

Low GI foods lead to a slower release of glucose into the bloodstream, which helps maintain more stable blood sugar levels. This is particularly beneficial for individuals with diabetes or insulin resistance, as it reduces the likelihood of sudden spikes and crashes in blood glucose levels.

2. Enhanced Satiety and Weight Management

Low glycemic foods tend to be more filling and provide longer-lasting satiety compared to their high glycemic counterparts. This can help control appetite and reduce overall calorie intake, making it easier to manage and maintain a healthy weight. Furthermore, a diet rich in low GI foods can reduce the risk of obesity, which is a significant risk factor for various chronic diseases.

Low GI foods tend to be more filling and provide longer-lasting satiety compared to high GI foods. This can help reduce overall calorie intake and support weight management efforts. By preventing rapid drops in blood sugar, low GI foods also minimize cravings and overeating.

3. Reduced Risk of Chronic Diseases

Consistently choosing low glycemic meals can have a positive impact on cardiovascular health. Studies have shown that low GI diets are associated with lower levels of LDL (bad) cholesterol and triglycerides, both of which are risk factors for heart disease. Additionally, the gradual release of glucose helps maintain healthy blood pressure levels.

Regular consumption of low GI foods is associated with a lower risk of developing chronic diseases such as heart disease, type 2 diabetes, and certain cancers. The steady supply of glucose helps reduce stress on the body's insulin response, lowering the risk of insulin resistance and related health issues.

4. Sustained Energy Levels

By providing a more gradual release of energy, low GI foods help maintain consistent energy levels throughout the day. This can improve overall physical and mental performance, making it easier to stay active and focused.

5. Better Diabetes Management

For individuals with diabetes, controlling blood sugar levels is critical. Low glycemic meals can help manage blood glucose levels more effectively, reducing the need for frequent adjustments in medication and lowering the risk of complications associated with diabetes. By choosing foods that have a minimal impact on blood sugar, people with diabetes can achieve better long-term control of their condition.

6. Enhanced Overall Health

Beyond the specific benefits related to blood sugar and weight management, low glycemic meals contribute to overall health and well-being. These meals often include a variety of nutrient-dense foods such as vegetables, fruits, whole grains, and legumes, which provide essential vitamins, minerals, and antioxidants. This balanced approach to eating supports immune function, digestive health, and energy production.

Remember, the GI is just one piece of the puzzle. Other factors like portion size, food combinations, and cooking methods can also influence your blood sugar response. This book will delve deeper into these aspects in the coming chapters.

Foods to eat on the low glycemic diet

When following a low glycemic diet, the focus is on choosing foods that have a minimal impact on blood sugar levels, promoting stable energy and better overall health. Here's a comprehensive list of foods to include in your low glycemic diet:

1. Non-Starchy Vegetables: Load up on colorful vegetables such as leafy greens, broccoli, cauliflower, bell peppers, tomatoes, cucumbers, zucchini, and carrots. These veggies are rich in fiber, vitamins, and minerals, and have a low glycemic index, making them excellent choices for maintaining stable blood sugar levels.

2. Whole Grains: Opt for whole grains such as oats, barley, quinoa, brown rice, and bulgur. These grains are packed with fiber, which slows down the absorption of glucose into the bloodstream, resulting in a lower glycemic response compared to refined grains like white rice and white bread.

3. Legumes: Incorporate beans, lentils, chickpeas, and peas into your meals. Legumes are high in fiber and protein, making them a nutritious and filling addition to soups, salads, stews, and casseroles. Plus, they have a low glycemic index, helping to stabilize blood sugar levels.

4. Lean Proteins: Include lean sources of protein such as skinless poultry, fish, tofu, tempeh, eggs, and low-fat dairy products. Protein-rich foods have minimal impact on blood sugar levels and help promote satiety, making them essential components of a low glycemic diet.

5. Healthy Fats: Incorporate sources of healthy fats such as avocados, nuts, seeds, and olive oil into your meals. These fats help slow down the digestion of carbohydrates, resulting in a lower glycemic response and prolonged feelings of fullness.

6. Fruits: Choose whole fruits such as berries, apples, oranges, pears, and kiwi, which have a lower glycemic index compared to tropical fruits like watermelon and pineapple. Enjoy fruits in moderation and pair them with protein or healthy fats to further mitigate their impact on blood sugar levels.

7. Dairy: Opt for low-fat or non-fat dairy products such as Greek yogurt, cottage cheese, and skim milk. Dairy products contain protein and calcium, which contribute to satiety and bone health. Choose plain or unsweetened varieties to avoid added sugars.

8. Herbs and Spices: Flavor your meals with herbs and spices such as garlic, ginger, cinnamon, turmeric, and chili powder. Not only do these add depth and complexity to your dishes, but some, like cinnamon, have been shown to help regulate blood sugar levels.

By incorporating these nutrient-dense, low glycemic foods into your diet, you can enjoy a wide variety of delicious meals while supporting stable blood sugar levels, optimal energy, and overall well-being. Remember to focus on whole, unprocessed foods and to balance your plate with a combination of carbohydrates, protein, and healthy fats for maximum health benefits.

The Glycemic Index is a powerful tool that can guide healthier dietary choices. By focusing on low glycemic foods, you can achieve better blood sugar control, manage your weight more effectively, reduce the risk of chronic diseases, and maintain consistent energy levels throughout the day. Understanding and applying the principles of the Glycemic Index is a crucial step towards a healthier, more balanced lifestyle.

Foods to avoid on the low glycemic diet

When following a low glycemic diet, it's important to be mindful of the foods that can cause blood sugar levels to spike quickly. Here's a detailed list of foods to avoid or limit:

1. Highly Processed Carbohydrates: Steer clear of highly processed carbohydrates such as white bread, white rice, sugary cereals, and pastries. These foods are rapidly digested and can cause a sharp increase in blood sugar levels.

2. Sugary Snacks and Sweets: Limit your intake of sugary snacks and sweets such as candy, cookies, cakes, and sweetened beverages. These items are packed with added sugars, which can lead to rapid fluctuations in blood sugar levels.

3. Sweetened Beverages: Avoid sugary drinks such as soda, fruit juices, energy drinks, and sweetened teas. These beverages contain large amounts of added sugars and offer little to no nutritional value.

4. Processed and Fried Foods: Cut back on processed and fried foods such as fast food, potato chips, French fries, and packaged snacks. These foods are often high in unhealthy fats, refined carbohydrates, and sodium, which can contribute to spikes in blood sugar and insulin levels.

5. White Potatoes: While potatoes can be a nutritious part of a balanced diet, white potatoes have a high glycemic index and can cause rapid increases in blood sugar levels. Opt for sweet potatoes or other root vegetables instead.

6. Highly Sweetened Breakfast Cereals: Choose breakfast cereals that are low in added sugars and high in fiber. Many commercial cereals are loaded with sugar, which can lead to blood sugar spikes and crashes later in the day.

7. Processed Meats: Limit your intake of processed meats such as bacon, sausage, hot dogs, and deli meats. These meats often contain added sugars, sodium, and preservatives, which can negatively impact blood sugar and overall health.

8. Desserts and Pastries: Indulge in desserts and pastries sparingly, as they are typically high in sugar, refined flour, and unhealthy fats. Opt for healthier alternatives such as fruit-based desserts or homemade treats made with whole grains and natural sweeteners.

By avoiding or limiting these high glycemic foods and focusing on whole, unprocessed options, you can better regulate your blood sugar levels and support overall health and well-being. Remember to read food labels carefully, prioritize nutrient-dense choices, and enjoy treats in moderation to maintain a balanced and sustainable low glycemic diet.

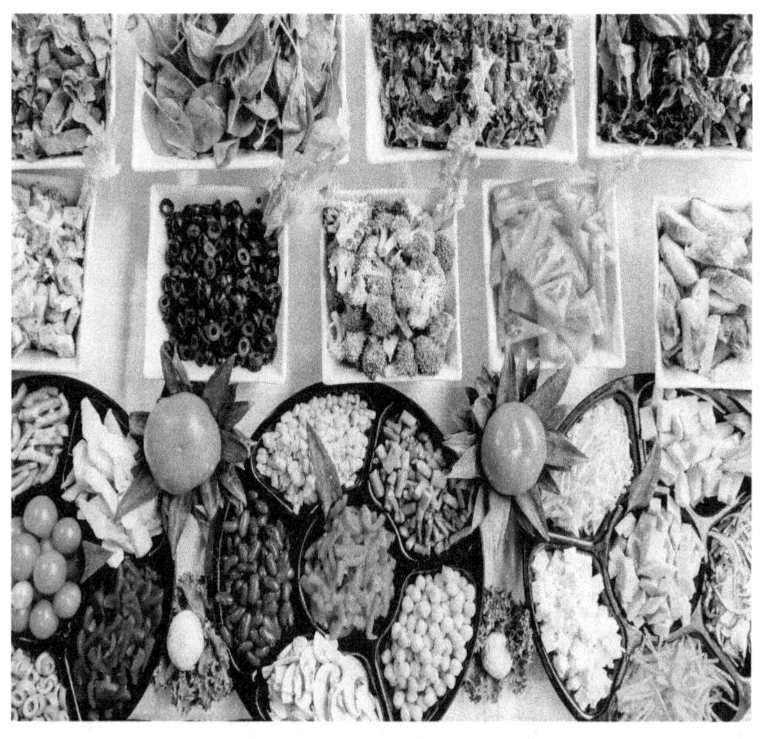

Chapter 2: Identifying Low Glycemic Foods

Knowing which foods have a low glycemic index (GI) can help you make better dietary choices that support your health goals. This chapter provides a detailed overview of low glycemic foods, how to identify them, and practical tips for incorporating them into your daily diet.

Understanding which foods fall into the category of low glycemic can be immensely helpful in crafting a diet that promotes stable blood sugar levels and overall health. In this chapter, we'll explore a variety of foods that are low on the glycemic index and discuss the factors that contribute to their classification.

1. Non-Starchy Vegetables:
Non-starchy vegetables are excellent choices for low glycemic eating. Non-starchy vegetables are generally low in GI and high in essential nutrients.
These include leafy greens like spinach, kale, and lettuce, as well as cruciferous vegetables such as broccoli, cauliflower, and Brussels sprouts. These vegetables are not only low in carbohydrates but also

rich in fiber, vitamins, and minerals, making them essential components of a balanced diet.

2. Legumes:

Legumes, such as lentils, chickpeas, and black beans, are another group of foods that are low on the glycemic index. These plant-based sources of protein and fiber provide a steady source of energy and promote feelings of fullness and satiety. Including legumes in your meals can help stabilize blood sugar levels and support overall health.

3. Whole Grains:

When it comes to grains, opting for whole grains over refined grains is key to maintaining a low glycemic diet. Whole grains like quinoa, barley, and brown rice are rich in fiber, which slows down digestion and helps prevent rapid spikes in blood sugar. These grains also offer a wide range of nutrients, including vitamins, minerals, and antioxidants, making them valuable additions to any meal.

4. Fruits:

While fruits contain natural sugars, many have a low GI due to their fiber content and other nutritional components.

While some fruits are higher on the glycemic index than others, many fruits can still be enjoyed as part of a low glycemic diet. Berries, such as strawberries, blueberries, and raspberries, are particularly low in sugar and high in fiber, making them excellent choices for keeping blood sugar levels in check. Other lower glycemic fruits include apples, pears, and citrus fruits like oranges and grapefruits.

5. Nuts and Seeds:
Nuts and seeds are nutrient-dense foods that are low in carbohydrates and high in healthy fats, protein, and fiber. Almonds, walnuts, chia seeds, and flaxseeds are all examples of low glycemic options that can be incorporated into snacks or meals to add texture, flavor, and nutritional value.

6. Dairy Products:
Many dairy products, such as plain yogurt and cheese, have a low glycemic index and can be included in a low glycemic diet in moderation. Opting for unsweetened varieties of yogurt and choosing cheeses that are lower in fat can help minimize the impact on blood sugar levels while still providing essential nutrients like calcium and protein.

By familiarizing yourself with these low glycemic foods and incorporating them into your meals and snacks, you can create a balanced and satisfying diet that supports stable blood sugar levels, sustained energy, and overall well-being. Experiment with different combinations and recipes to discover delicious ways to enjoy these nutritious foods while reaping the benefits of low glycemic eating.

Characteristics of Low Glycemic Foods

Low glycemic foods generally share certain characteristics that contribute to their slow digestion and gradual impact on blood sugar levels.

When it comes to identifying low glycemic foods, several key characteristics set them apart from their high glycemic counterparts. Understanding these characteristics can help you make informed choices about the foods you include in your diet and ensure that you're prioritizing options that promote stable blood sugar levels and overall health. Let's explore some of the defining features of low glycemic foods:

1. High in Fiber:

Low glycemic foods are typically rich in dietary fiber, which plays a crucial role in slowing down the digestion and absorption of carbohydrates. This slow digestion process helps prevent rapid spikes in blood sugar levels, promoting more stable energy levels and reducing the risk of insulin resistance. Fiber also contributes to feelings of fullness and satiety, making low glycemic foods satisfying choices for meals and snacks.

2. Complex Carbohydrates:

Unlike high glycemic foods, which are often made with refined carbohydrates that are quickly broken down into sugar, low glycemic foods are composed of complex carbohydrates. These carbohydrates are found in whole, unprocessed foods such as whole grains, legumes, and vegetables. Because they contain more fiber, vitamins, and minerals than refined carbohydrates, complex carbohydrates provide a more sustained source of energy and have less of an impact on blood sugar levels.

3. Minimal Processing:

Low glycemic foods are generally minimally processed or in their natural state. Processing can strip foods of their fiber and nutrients, leading to faster digestion and absorption of carbohydrates and ultimately higher glycemic responses. By choosing whole, unprocessed foods whenever possible, you can ensure that you're consuming low glycemic options that support optimal health and well-being.

4. Low in Added Sugars:

Added sugars are a hallmark of high glycemic foods, as they contribute to rapid spikes in blood sugar levels when consumed in excess. In contrast, low glycemic foods are typically low in added sugars or contain natural sugars that are accompanied by fiber and other nutrients. Choosing foods with minimal added sugars, such as plain yogurt, unsweetened oatmeal, and fresh fruits, can help keep blood sugar levels stable and promote better overall health.

5. Rich in Nutrients:

Low glycemic foods are not only low in sugar but also rich in essential nutrients like vitamins, minerals, and antioxidants. These nutrients are vital for supporting various bodily functions and promoting overall health and vitality. By prioritizing nutrient-dense foods like fruits, vegetables, whole grains, and lean proteins, you can ensure that your diet is not only low glycemic but also nutritionally balanced and beneficial for long-term health.

Incorporating these characteristics into your food choices can help you create a diet that is low on the glycemic index and high in nutritional value. By focusing on fiber-rich, minimally processed, and nutrient-dense foods, you can enjoy stable energy levels, better blood sugar control, and improved overall well-being.

Practical Tips for Incorporating Low Glycemic Foods

Incorporating low glycemic foods into your diet doesn't have to be complicated. With a few simple strategies and practical tips, you can make low glycemic eating a seamless part of your daily routine. Here are some practical suggestions to help you get started:

1. Start with Whole Foods:

Focus on incorporating whole, unprocessed foods into your meals and snacks. Choose fresh fruits and vegetables, whole grains, lean proteins, and healthy fats as the foundation of your diet. These foods are naturally low on the glycemic index and provide a wealth of nutrients to support your overall health and well-being.

2. Read Labels Wisely:

When shopping for packaged foods, take the time to read nutrition labels and ingredient lists carefully. Look for products that are low in added sugars, refined carbohydrates, and unhealthy fats. Pay attention to the serving size and the glycemic load of the food, which takes into account both the quantity and quality of carbohydrates.

3. Balance Your Plate:

Aim to create balanced meals that include a combination of carbohydrates, protein, and healthy fats. This balance helps slow down the digestion and absorption of carbohydrates, leading to more stable blood sugar levels. For example, pair a serving of whole grains with lean protein and a generous portion of vegetables for a satisfying and nutritious meal.

4. Experiment with Cooking Methods:

Explore different cooking methods that can help lower the glycemic index of foods. For example, steaming, roasting, and grilling vegetables can enhance their flavor and texture without adding extra fats or sugars. Similarly, cooking grains such as quinoa or barley with a little bit of fat and protein can help slow down their digestion and reduce their glycemic impact.

5. Snack Smart:

Choose low glycemic snacks to keep hunger at bay between meals. Opt for options like raw vegetables with hummus, Greek yogurt with berries, or a small handful of nuts and seeds. These snacks provide a satisfying combination of fiber, protein, and healthy fats to help keep you full and energized throughout the day.

6. Plan Ahead:

Take the time to plan your meals and snacks in advance to ensure that you have plenty of low glycemic options on hand. Stock your pantry and refrigerator with nutritious staples like whole grains, legumes, fruits, and vegetables, so you always have healthy choices available when hunger strikes.

7. Be Mindful of Portion Sizes:

While low glycemic foods are beneficial for stabilizing blood sugar levels, portion control is still important. Pay attention to serving sizes and avoid overeating, even if the food is considered low glycemic. Eating balanced meals and snacks in moderation is key to maintaining a healthy diet and achieving your wellness goals.

By incorporating these practical tips into your daily routine, you can effortlessly integrate low glycemic foods into your diet and enjoy the many health benefits they have to offer. With a little bit of planning and creativity, you can create delicious and nutritious meals that support your overall well-being for the long term.

Sample Low Glycemic Meals

Here are some ideas for meals that are both delicious and low in glycemic index:

Breakfast

Overnight Chia Pudding

- **Ingredients:** Chia seeds, almond milk, vanilla extract, fresh berries
- **Instructions:** Mix chia seeds with almond milk and a splash of vanilla extract. Refrigerate overnight. Top with fresh berries in the morning.

Lunch

Quinoa and Black Bean Salad

- **Ingredients:** Cooked quinoa, black beans, cherry tomatoes, cucumber, red onion, lime juice, olive oil, cilantro

- **Instructions:** Combine all ingredients in a bowl. Drizzle with lime juice and olive oil. Toss gently and serve.

Dinner

Baked Salmon with Vegetables

- **Ingredients:** Salmon fillets, broccoli, carrots, olive oil, lemon, garlic, herbs
- **Instructions:** Place salmon and vegetables on a baking sheet. Drizzle with olive oil and lemon juice, add minced garlic and herbs. Bake at 375°F (190°C) for 20-25 minutes.

Snacks

Apple Slices with Almond Butter

- **Ingredients:** Apple, almond butter
- **Instructions:** Slice the apple and serve with a side of almond butter for dipping.

Hummus with Vegetable Sticks

- **Ingredients:** Hummus, carrot sticks, celery sticks, bell pepper strips
- **Instructions:** Serve hummus with an assortment of fresh vegetable sticks.

Identifying and incorporating low glycemic foods into your diet is a practical and effective way to manage blood sugar levels, enhance satiety, and improve overall health. By focusing on whole, fiber-rich foods and balancing your meals, you can enjoy a variety of delicious and nutritious options that support a low glycemic lifestyle. This approach not only benefits individuals managing conditions like diabetes but also promotes long-term health and well-being for everyone.

By following these practical tips and strategies, you can create a low glycemic meal plan that supports your health goals and enhances your overall well-being. With careful planning, balanced meals, and a commitment to listening to your body, you can enjoy the many benefits of low glycemic eating and feel your best both inside and out.

Chapter 3: Healthy and Nutritious Low Glycemic Breakfast Recipes

Creating delicious, low glycemic meals can be both enjoyable and rewarding. This chapter provides a variety of recipes for breakfast, lunch, dinner, and snacks, all designed to keep your blood sugar levels stable while providing essential nutrients and satisfying flavors.

1. Spinach and Feta Egg Muffins

Ingredients:
- 6 large eggs
- 1 cup fresh spinach, chopped
- 1/2 cup feta cheese, crumbled
- 1/4 cup diced tomatoes
- Salt and pepper to taste

Instructions:
1. Preheat the oven to 350°F (175°C).

2. In a bowl, whisk the eggs, then stir in spinach, feta, and tomatoes.
3. Season with salt and pepper.
4. Pour mixture into a greased muffin tin.
5. Bake for 20-25 minutes, until eggs are set.

2. Avocado Toast with Poached Egg

Ingredients:
- 1 slice whole grain bread
- 1/2 avocado, mashed
- 1 large egg
- Salt, pepper, and red pepper flakes to taste

Instructions:
1. Toast the bread.
2. Spread mashed avocado on the toast.
3. Poach the egg and place it on top of the avocado.
4. Season with salt, pepper, and red pepper flakes.

3. Berry Smoothie Bowl

Ingredients:
- 1 cup frozen mixed berries
- 1/2 banana
- 1/2 cup unsweetened almond milk
- 1/4 cup Greek yogurt
- 1 tbsp chia seeds

- 1 tbsp granola (optional)

Instructions:
1. Blend berries, banana, almond milk, and Greek yogurt until smooth.
2. Pour into a bowl and top with chia seeds and granola.

4. Oatmeal with Almonds and Berries

Ingredients:
- 1/2 cup steel-cut oats
- 1 cup water or unsweetened almond milk
- 1/4 cup fresh berries
- 1 tbsp sliced almonds
- 1 tsp honey (optional)

Instructions:
1. Cook oats in water or almond milk according to package instructions.
2. Top with fresh berries, almonds, and a drizzle of honey.

5. Greek Yogurt Parfait

Ingredients:
- 1 cup plain Greek yogurt
- 1/2 cup granola
- 1/2 cup mixed berries

- 1 tbsp honey (optional)

Instructions:
1. Layer Greek yogurt, granola, and berries in a glass or bowl.
2. Drizzle with honey if desired.

6. Sweet Potato and Black Bean Breakfast Burrito

Ingredients:
- 1 small sweet potato, diced and roasted
- 1/2 cup black beans, drained and rinsed
- 1 whole grain tortilla
- 2 tbsp salsa
- 1 tbsp shredded cheese

Instructions:
1. Warm the tortilla and fill with sweet potato, black beans, salsa, and cheese.
2. Roll up and enjoy.

7. Cottage Cheese and Fruit

Ingredients:
- 1 cup cottage cheese
- 1/2 cup sliced peaches or berries
- 1 tbsp chia seeds

Instructions:

1. Top cottage cheese with fruit and chia seeds.

8. Banana and Almond Butter Smoothie

Ingredients:
- 1 banana
- 1 tbsp almond butter
- 1 cup unsweetened almond milk
- 1 tbsp chia seeds
- 1 tsp honey (optional)

Instructions:
1. Blend all ingredients until smooth.
2. Serve immediately.

9. Quinoa Breakfast Bowl

Ingredients:
- 1/2 cup cooked quinoa
- 1/4 cup Greek yogurt
- 1/4 cup fresh berries
- 1 tbsp honey or maple syrup

Instructions:
1. Mix quinoa with Greek yogurt.
2. Top with fresh berries and a drizzle of honey or maple syrup.

10. Mushroom and Spinach Breakfast Skillet

Ingredients:
- 1 cup sliced mushrooms
- 1 cup fresh spinach
- 2 large eggs
- 1 tbsp olive oil
- Salt and pepper to taste

Instructions:
1. Heat up some olive oil in a skillet over medium heat.
2. Sauté mushrooms until tender, then add spinach and cook until wilted.
3. Create two small wells and crack an egg into each.
4. Cover and cook until eggs are set.
5. Season with salt and pepper.

11. Chia Seed Pudding with Mango

Ingredients:
- 1/4 cup chia seeds
- 1 cup coconut milk
- 1/2 cup diced mango
- 1 tsp honey (optional)

Instructions:

1. Mix chia seeds and coconut milk, refrigerate overnight.

2. Top with diced mango and a drizzle of honey.

12. Zucchini and Tomato Frittata

Ingredients:
- 6 large eggs
- 1 cup zucchini, grated
- 1/2 cup diced tomatoes
- 1/4 cup feta cheese, crumbled
- Salt and pepper to taste

Instructions:
1. Preheat the oven to 350°F (175°C).
2. Whisk eggs and stir in zucchini, tomatoes, and feta.
3. Season with salt and pepper.
4. Pour into a greased baking dish and bake for 20-25 minutes.

13. Almond Flour Pancakes

Ingredients:
- 1 cup almond flour
- 2 large eggs
- 1/4 cup unsweetened almond milk
- 1 tsp baking powder
- 1 tsp vanilla extract

- 1 tbsp honey (optional)

Instructions:
1. Mix all ingredients until smooth.
2. Cook pancakes on a non-stick skillet over medium heat.
3. Serve with fresh berries and a drizzle of honey.

14. Blueberry and Spinach Smoothie

Ingredients:
- 1 cup fresh spinach
- 1 cup frozen blueberries
- 1/2 banana
- 1 cup unsweetened almond milk
- 1 tbsp chia seeds

Instructions:
1. Blend all ingredients until smooth.
2. Serve immediately.

15. Breakfast Burrito with Avocado and Egg

Ingredients:
- 1 whole grain tortilla
- 1/2 avocado, sliced
- 2 scrambled eggs
- 1/4 cup black beans

- Salsa to taste

Instructions:
1. Warm the tortilla and fill with avocado, scrambled eggs, black beans, and salsa.
2. Roll up and enjoy.

16. Peanut Butter Banana Toast

Ingredients:
- 1 slice whole grain bread
- 1 tbsp natural peanut butter
- 1/2 banana, sliced

Instructions:
1. Toast the bread.
2. Spread some peanut butter on the toast and then add slices of banana on top.

17. Coconut Flour Waffles

Ingredients:
- 1/2 cup coconut flour
- 3 large eggs
- 1/4 cup coconut milk
- 1 tsp vanilla extract
- 1 tbsp honey (optional)

Instructions:
1. Mix all ingredients until smooth.
2. Cook in a preheated waffle iron.
3. Serve with fresh fruit.

18. Apple Cinnamon Oatmeal

Ingredients:
- 1/2 cup rolled oats
- 1 cup water or unsweetened almond milk
- 1/2 apple, diced
- 1/2 tsp cinnamon
- 1 tbsp chopped walnuts

Instructions:
1. Cook oats in water or almond milk.
2. Stir in apple and cinnamon.
3. Top with chopped walnuts.

19. Spinach and Avocado Smoothie

Ingredients:
- 1 cup fresh spinach
- 1/2 avocado
- 1/2 banana
- 1 cup unsweetened almond milk
- 1 tsp honey (optional)

Instructions:

1. Blend all ingredients until smooth.
2. Serve immediately.

20. Cottage Cheese with Pineapple

Ingredients:
- 1 cup cottage cheese
- 1/2 cup diced pineapple
- 1 tbsp chia seeds

Instructions:

1. Top cottage cheese with pineapple and chia seeds.

21. Tomato and Basil Frittata

Ingredients:
- 6 large eggs
- 1/2 cup diced tomatoes
- 1/4 cup fresh basil, chopped
- 1/4 cup mozzarella cheese, shredded
- Salt and pepper to taste

Instructions:

1. Preheat the oven to 350°F (175°C).
2. Whisk eggs and stir in tomatoes, basil, and mozzarella.
3. Season with salt and pepper.

4. Pour into a greased baking dish and bake for 20-25 minutes.

22. Strawberry Chia Seed Smoothie

Ingredients:
- 1 cup fresh strawberries
- 1/2 banana
- 1 cup unsweetened almond milk
- 1 tbsp chia seeds

Instructions:
1. Blend all ingredients until smooth.
2. Serve immediately.

23. Mushroom and Spinach Breakfast Quesadilla

Ingredients:
- 1 whole grain tortilla
- 1/2 cup sliced mushrooms
- 1 cup fresh spinach
- 1/4 cup shredded cheese
- 1 tbsp olive oil

Instructions:
1. Sauté mushrooms and spinach in olive oil until tender.
2. Place on one half of the tortilla, sprinkle with cheese, and fold.

3. Cook in a skillet until the tortilla is crispy and the cheese is melted.

24. Chia Seed Pancakes

Ingredients:
- 1/2 cup almond flour
- 1/4 cup chia seeds
- 2 large eggs
- 1/4 cup unsweetened almond milk
- 1 tsp baking powder
- 1 tsp vanilla extract

Instructions:
1. Mix all ingredients until smooth.
2. Cook pancakes on a non-stick skillet over medium heat.
3. Serve with fresh berries.

25. Savory Oatmeal with Spinach and Poached Egg

Ingredients:
- 1/2 cup rolled oats
- 1 cup water or unsweetened almond milk
- 1 cup fresh spinach
- 1 large egg
- Salt and pepper to taste

Instructions:

1. Cook oats in water or almond milk.

2. Stir in fresh spinach until wilted.

3. Top with a poached egg and season with salt and pepper.

26. Coconut and Berry Smoothie

Ingredients:
- 1/2 cup frozen mixed berries
- 1/2 cup coconut milk
- 1/2 banana
- 1 tbsp chia seeds

Instructions:

1. Blend all ingredients until smooth.

2. Serve immediately.

27. Avocado and Tomato Toast

Ingredients:
- 1 slice whole grain bread
- 1/2 avocado, mashed
- 1/2 tomato, sliced
- Salt and pepper to taste

Instructions:

1. Toast the bread.

2. Spread mashed avocado on the toast and top with tomato slices.

3. Season with salt and pepper.

28. Buckwheat Pancakes

Ingredients:
- 1 cup buckwheat flour
- 2 large eggs
- 1/2 cup unsweetened almond milk
- 1 tsp baking powder
- 1 tbsp honey (optional)

Instructions:

1. Mix all ingredients until smooth.

2. Cook pancakes on a non-stick skillet over medium heat.

3. Serve with fresh fruit.

29. Mango and Coconut Chia Pudding

Ingredients:
- 1/4 cup chia seeds
- 1 cup coconut milk
- 1/2 cup diced mango
- 1 tsp honey (optional)

Instructions:

1. Mix chia seeds and coconut milk, refrigerate overnight.
2. Top with diced mango and a drizzle of honey.

30. Pumpkin Spice Smoothie

Ingredients:
- 1/2 cup pumpkin puree
- 1/2 banana
- 1 cup unsweetened almond milk
- 1 tsp pumpkin pie spice
- 1 tbsp chia seeds

Instructions:
1. Blend all ingredients until smooth.
2. Serve immediately.

31. Cauliflower Hash Browns

Ingredients:
- 2 cups grated cauliflower
- 2 large eggs
- 1/4 cup grated Parmesan cheese
- 1/4 cup chopped green onions
- Salt and pepper to taste

Instructions:
1. Preheat the oven to 400°F (200°C).

2. Mix all ingredients in a bowl.

3. Form into patties and place on a baking sheet lined with parchment paper.

4. Bake for 20-25 minutes until golden brown.

32. Avocado and Cottage Cheese Toast

Ingredients:
- 1 slice whole grain bread
- 1/2 avocado, sliced
- 1/2 cup cottage cheese
- Salt and pepper to taste

Instructions:
1. Toast the bread.
2. Top with cottage cheese and avocado slices.
3. Season with salt and pepper.

33. Sweet Potato and Kale Hash

Ingredients:
- 1 large sweet potato, diced
- 2 cups chopped kale
- 1 small onion, diced
- 1 tbsp olive oil
- Salt and pepper to taste

Instructions:

1. Heat up some olive oil in a skillet over medium heat.
2. Add sweet potato and onion, cook until tender.
3. Add kale and cook until wilted.
4. Season with salt and pepper.

34. Almond Butter and Berry Smoothie

Ingredients:
- 1 cup unsweetened almond milk
- 1/2 cup frozen mixed berries
- 1 tbsp almond butter
- 1/2 banana
- 1 tbsp chia seeds

Instructions:
1. Blend all ingredients until smooth.
2. Serve immediately.

35. Quinoa and Berry Breakfast Bowl

Ingredients:
- 1/2 cup cooked quinoa
- 1/2 cup mixed berries
- 1/4 cup Greek yogurt
- 1 tbsp chia seeds

Instructions:
1. Mix quinoa with Greek yogurt.

2. Top with berries and chia seeds.

36. Broccoli and Cheese Omelette

Ingredients:
- 3 large eggs
- 1/2 cup steamed broccoli, chopped
- 1/4 cup shredded cheese
- Salt and pepper to taste
- 1 tbsp olive oil

Instructions:
1. Whisk eggs in a bowl and season with salt and pepper.
2. Heat olive oil in a skillet over medium heat.
3. Add eggs, then sprinkle broccoli and cheese over the top.
4. Cook until eggs are set, folding in half.

37. Coconut Flour Banana Muffins

Ingredients:
- 1 cup coconut flour
- 2 large eggs
- 1/2 cup mashed banana
- 1/4 cup coconut milk
- 1 tsp baking powder
- 1 tsp vanilla extract

Instructions:
1. Preheat the oven to 350°F (175°C).
2. Mix all ingredients until smooth.
3. Pour into muffin tins and bake for 20-25 minutes.

38. Smoked Salmon and Avocado Toast

Ingredients:
- 1 slice whole grain bread
- 1/4 avocado, sliced
- 2 oz smoked salmon
- 1 tsp lemon juice
- Salt and pepper to taste

Instructions:
1. Toast the bread.
2. Top with avocado slices, smoked salmon, and a drizzle of lemon juice.
3. Season with salt and pepper.

39. Berry and Spinach Smoothie

Ingredients:
- 1 cup fresh spinach
- 1 cup frozen mixed berries
- 1/2 banana
- 1 cup unsweetened almond milk
- 1 tbsp chia seeds

Instructions:
1. Blend all ingredients until smooth.
2. Serve immediately.

40. Zucchini and Egg Muffins

Ingredients:
- 1 cup grated zucchini
- 6 large eggs
- 1/4 cup grated Parmesan cheese
- 1/4 cup diced tomatoes
- Salt and pepper to taste

Instructions:
1. Preheat the oven to 350°F (175°C).
2. Mix all ingredients in a bowl.
3. Pour into a greased muffin tin.
4. Bake for 20-25 minutes, until eggs are set.

41. Almond Flour Waffles

Ingredients:
- 1 cup almond flour
- 2 large eggs
- 1/4 cup unsweetened almond milk
- 1 tsp baking powder
- 1 tsp vanilla extract

Instructions:

1. Mix all ingredients until smooth.
2. Cook in a preheated waffle iron.
3. Serve with fresh fruit.

42. Peanut Butter and Berry Smoothie

Ingredients:

- 1 cup unsweetened almond milk
- 1/2 cup frozen mixed berries
- 1 tbsp peanut butter
- 1/2 banana
- 1 tbsp chia seeds

Instructions:

1. Blend all ingredients until smooth.
2. Serve immediately.

43. Sweet Potato Breakfast Bowl

Ingredients:

- 1 large sweet potato, diced and roasted
- 1/2 cup black beans, drained and rinsed
- 1/4 cup diced avocado
- 2 tbsp salsa

Instructions:

1. Roast sweet potato until tender.
2. Combine with black beans and avocado in a bowl.
3. Top with salsa.

44. Cottage Cheese and Berry Parfait

Ingredients:
- 1 cup cottage cheese
- 1/2 cup mixed berries
- 1 tbsp chia seeds
- 1 tbsp honey (optional)

Instructions:

1. Layer cottage cheese, berries, and chia seeds in a glass or bowl.
2. Drizzle with honey if desired.

45. Tomato and Avocado Omelette

Ingredients:
- 3 large eggs
- 1/2 avocado, diced
- 1/2 cup diced tomatoes
- Salt and pepper to taste
- 1 tbsp olive oil

Instructions:
1. Whisk eggs in a bowl and season with salt and pepper.
2. Heat up some olive oil in a skillet over medium heat.
3. Add eggs, then sprinkle avocado and tomatoes over the top.
4. Cook until eggs are set, folding in half.

46. Coconut Flour and Blueberry Muffins

Ingredients:
- 1 cup coconut flour
- 2 large eggs
- 1/2 cup coconut milk
- 1/2 cup fresh blueberries
- 1 tsp baking powder
- 1 tsp vanilla extract

Instructions:
1. Preheat the oven to 350°F (175°C).
2. Mix all ingredients until smooth.
3. Fold in blueberries.
4. Pour into muffin tins and bake for 20-25 minutes.

47. Avocado and Spinach Smoothie

Ingredients:
- 1 cup fresh spinach
- 1/2 avocado

- 1/2 banana
- 1 cup unsweetened almond milk
- 1 tbsp chia seeds

Instructions:
1. Blend all ingredients until smooth.
2. Serve immediately.

48. Sweet Potato and Black Bean Breakfast Burrito

Ingredients:
- 1 whole grain tortilla
- 1/2 cup roasted sweet potato
- 1/4 cup black beans, drained and rinsed
- 1 tbsp salsa
- 1 tbsp shredded cheese

Instructions:
1. Warm the tortilla.
2. Fill with sweet potato, black beans, salsa, and cheese.
3. Roll up and enjoy.

49. Cottage Cheese with Apple and Cinnamon

Ingredients:
- 1 cup cottage cheese
- 1/2 apple, diced
- 1/2 tsp cinnamon

- 1 tbsp chopped walnuts

Instructions:
1. Top cottage cheese with apple, cinnamon, and walnuts.

50. Pumpkin and Chia Seed Pudding

Ingredients:
- 1/4 cup chia seeds
- 1 cup unsweetened almond milk
- 1/4 cup pumpkin puree
- 1 tsp pumpkin pie spice

Instructions:
1. Mix chia seeds, almond milk, pumpkin puree, and pumpkin pie spice.
2. Refrigerate overnight.
3. Serve chilled.

51. Broccoli and Cheddar Breakfast Casserole

Ingredients:
- 2 cups broccoli florets, steamed
- 6 large eggs
- 1 cup shredded cheddar cheese
- Salt and pepper to taste

Instructions:

1. Preheat the oven to 350°F (175°C).

2. Mix eggs, broccoli, and cheddar in a bowl.

3. Season with salt and pepper.

4. Pour into a greased baking dish and bake for 25-30 minutes.

52. Berry and Spinach Breakfast Wrap

Ingredients:

- 1 whole grain tortilla
- 1/2 cup fresh spinach
- 1/2 cup mixed berries
- 1 tbsp almond butter

Instructions:

1. Spread almond butter on the tortilla.

2. Top with spinach and berries.

3. Roll up and enjoy.

53. Greek Yogurt and Mango Smoothie

Ingredients:

- 1 cup plain Greek yogurt
- 1/2 cup diced mango
- 1/2 banana
- 1 cup unsweetened almond milk
- 1 tbsp chia seeds

Instructions:

1. Blend all ingredients until smooth.
2. Serve immediately.

54. Savory Oatmeal with Mushrooms and Spinach

Ingredients:
- 1/2 cup rolled oats
- 1 cup water or unsweetened almond milk
- 1/2 cup sliced mushrooms
- 1 cup fresh spinach
- 1 tbsp olive oil
- Salt and pepper to taste

Instructions:

1. Cook oats in water or almond milk.
2. Sauté mushrooms and spinach in olive oil.
3. Stir into oatmeal and season with salt and pepper.

55. Zucchini and Tomato Breakfast Casserole

Ingredients:
- 1 cup grated zucchini
- 1/2 cup diced tomatoes
- 6 large eggs
- 1/4 cup grated Parmesan cheese
- Salt and pepper to taste

Instructions:
1. Preheat the oven to 350°F (175°C).
2. Mix all ingredients in a bowl.
3. Pour into a greased baking dish and bake for 25-30 minutes.

56. Almond Butter and Banana Smoothie

Ingredients:
- 1 cup unsweetened almond milk
- 1 banana
- 1 tbsp almond butter
- 1 tbsp chia seeds

Instructions:
1. Blend all ingredients until smooth.
2. Serve immediately.

57. Sweet Potato and Kale Breakfast Skillet

Ingredients:
- 1 large sweet potato, diced
- 2 cups chopped kale
- 1 small onion, diced
- 1 tbsp olive oil
- Salt and pepper to taste

Instructions:

1. Heat up some olive oil in a skillet over medium heat.
2. Add sweet potato and onion, cook until tender.
3. Add kale and cook until wilted.
4. Season with salt and pepper.

58. Cottage Cheese and Berry Breakfast Bowl

Ingredients:
- 1 cup cottage cheese
- 1/2 cup mixed berries
- 1 tbsp chia seeds

Instructions:
1. Top cottage cheese with berries and chia seeds.

59. Avocado and Egg Breakfast Wrap

Ingredients:
- 1 whole grain tortilla
- 1/2 avocado, sliced
- 2 scrambled eggs
- Salsa to taste

Instructions:
1. Warm the tortilla.
2. Fill with avocado, scrambled eggs, and salsa.
3. Roll up and enjoy.

60. Coconut Flour and Chocolate Chip Pancakes

Ingredients:
- 1 cup coconut flour
- 2 large eggs
- 1/4 cup coconut milk
- 1/4 cup dark chocolate chips
- 1 tsp baking powder
- 1 tsp vanilla extract

Instructions:
1. Mix all ingredients until smooth.
2. Cook pancakes on a non-stick skillet over medium heat.
3. Serve with fresh fruit.

61. Pumpkin and Spinach Smoothie

Ingredients:
- 1 cup fresh spinach
- 1/2 cup pumpkin puree
- 1/2 banana
- 1 cup unsweetened almond milk
- 1 tbsp chia seeds

Instructions:
1. Blend all ingredients until smooth.

2. Serve immediately.

62. Tomato and Basil Breakfast Wrap

Ingredients:
- 1 whole grain tortilla
- 1/2 cup diced tomatoes
- 1/4 cup fresh basil, chopped
- 1/4 cup shredded mozzarella cheese

Instructions:
1. Warm the tortilla.
2. Fill with tomatoes, basil, and mozzarella.
3. Roll up and enjoy.

63. Greek Yogurt and Strawberry Smoothie

Ingredients:
- 1 cup plain Greek yogurt
- 1/2 cup fresh strawberries
- 1/2 banana
- 1 cup unsweetened almond milk
- 1 tbsp chia seeds

Instructions:
1. Blend all ingredients until smooth.
2. Serve immediately.

64. Savory Oatmeal with Avocado and Egg

Ingredients:
- 1/2 cup rolled oats
- 1 cup water or unsweetened almond milk
- 1/2 avocado, diced
- 1 large egg
- Salt and pepper to taste

Instructions:
1. Cook oats in water or almond milk.
2. Stir in avocado.
3. Top with a poached egg and season with salt and pepper.

65. Zucchini and Mushroom Breakfast Casserole

Ingredients:
- 1 cup grated zucchini
- 1/2 cup sliced mushrooms
- 6 large eggs
- 1/4 cup grated Parmesan cheese
- Salt and pepper to taste

Instructions:
1. Preheat the oven to 350°F (175°C).
2. Mix all ingredients in a bowl.

3. Pour into a greased baking dish and bake for 25-30 minutes.

66. Almond Butter and Blueberry Smoothie

Ingredients:
- 1 cup unsweetened almond milk
- 1/2 cup fresh blueberries
- 1 tbsp almond butter
- 1/2 banana
- 1 tbsp chia seeds

Instructions:
1. Blend all ingredients until smooth.
2. Serve immediately.

67. Sweet Potato and Black Bean Breakfast Bowl

Ingredients:
- 1 large sweet potato, diced and roasted
- 1/2 cup black beans, drained and rinsed
- 1/4 cup diced avocado
- 2 tbsp salsa

Instructions:
1. Roast sweet potato until tender.
2. Combine with black beans and avocado in a bowl.
3. Top with salsa.

68. Cottage Cheese and Pineapple Parfait

Ingredients:
- 1 cup cottage cheese
- 1/2 cup diced pineapple
- 1 tbsp chia seeds
- 1 tbsp honey (optional)

Instructions:
1. Layer cottage cheese, pineapple, and chia seeds in a glass or bowl.
2. Drizzle with honey if desired.

69. Tomato and Spinach Omelette

Ingredients:
- 3 large eggs
- 1/2 cup diced tomatoes
- 1/2 cup fresh spinach
- Salt and pepper to taste
- 1 tbsp olive oil

Instructions:
1. Whisk eggs in a bowl and season with salt and pepper.
2. Heat up some olive oil in a skillet over medium heat.
3. Add eggs, then sprinkle tomatoes and spinach over the top.

4. Cook until eggs are set, folding in half.

70. Overnight Chia Pudding

Ingredients:
- 1/4 cup chia seeds
- 1 cup unsweetened almond milk
- 1 tsp vanilla extract
- 1/2 cup fresh berries (strawberries, blueberries, or raspberries)
- 1 tbsp honey or maple syrup (optional)

Instructions:
1. In a bowl, mix chia seeds, almond milk, and vanilla extract.
2. Stir well to combine and refrigerate overnight.
3. In the morning, give the pudding a good stir and top with fresh berries and a drizzle of honey or maple syrup if desired.

These recipes provide a diverse array of options to keep your breakfast routine exciting while maintaining low glycemic principles. Enjoy experimenting with these recipes to find your favorites and start your day with nutritious, satisfying meals.

Crafting low glycemic meals can be both easy and enjoyable with a variety of delicious recipes at your disposal. By focusing on whole foods, balancing macronutrients, and incorporating high-fiber ingredients, you can create meals that support stable blood sugar levels and overall health. These recipes offer a starting point for integrating low glycemic foods into your daily routine, providing flavorful and nutritious options for every meal of the day.

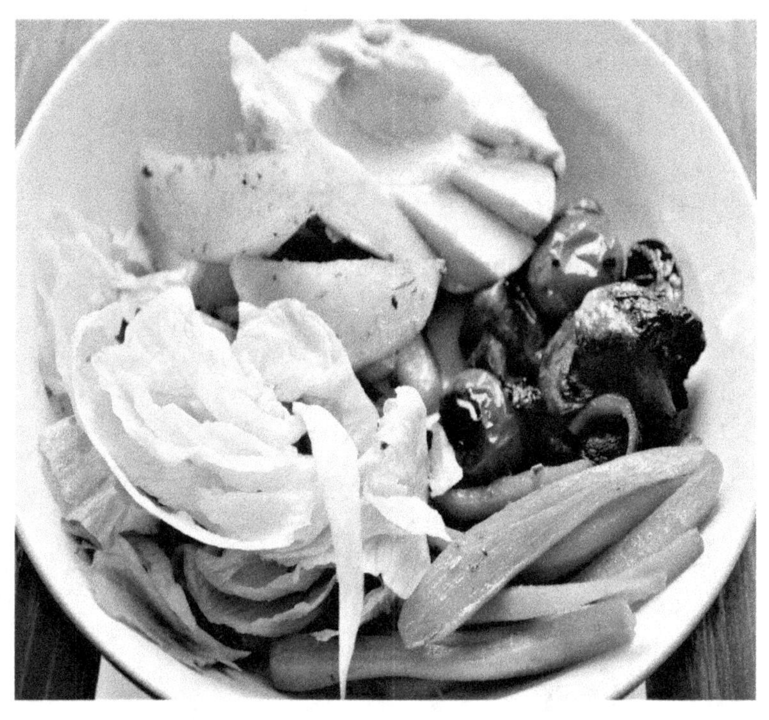

Chapter 4: Nutrient-Dense Low Glycemic Lunch Recipes

1. Quinoa and Black Bean Salad

Ingredients:
- 1 cup cooked quinoa
- 1 cup black beans, drained and rinsed
- 1 cup cherry tomatoes, halved
- 1/2 cup corn kernels
- 1/4 cup chopped cilantro
- 1/4 cup lime juice
- 1 tbsp olive oil
- Salt and pepper to taste

Instructions:
1. In a large bowl, combine quinoa, black beans, cherry tomatoes, corn, and cilantro.
2. In a small bowl, whisk together lime juice, olive oil, salt, and pepper.
3. Pour the dressing over the salad and toss to coat.

2. Grilled Chicken and Avocado Wrap

Ingredients:

- 1 whole grain tortilla
- 1/2 grilled chicken breast, sliced
- 1/2 avocado, sliced
- 1/4 cup shredded lettuce
- 1 tbsp Greek yogurt
- 1 tsp lime juice
- Salt and pepper to taste

Instructions:

1. Spread Greek yogurt on the tortilla.
2. Layer with grilled chicken, avocado, and lettuce.
3. Drizzle with lime juice and season with salt and pepper.
4. Roll up the tortilla and slice in half.

3. Lentil and Spinach Soup

Ingredients:

- 1 cup dried lentils
- 6 cups vegetable broth
- 1 onion, chopped
- 2 carrots, diced
- 2 celery stalks, diced
- 3 cups fresh spinach
- 2 cloves garlic, minced
- 1 tsp cumin
- Salt and pepper to taste

Instructions:

1. In a large pot, sauté onion, carrots, celery, and garlic until tender.
2. Add lentils, vegetable broth, and cumin.
3. Bring to a boil, then immediately reduce the heat and continue to simmer for twenty to twenty-five minutes.
4. Stir in spinach until wilted.
5. Season with salt and pepper.

4. Turkey and Veggie Lettuce Wraps

Ingredients:
- 1 cup cooked ground turkey
- 1/2 cup diced bell peppers
- 1/2 cup diced cucumbers
- 1/4 cup shredded carrots
- 1/4 cup hoisin sauce
- 8 large lettuce leaves

Instructions:

1. In a large bowl, combine cooked turkey, bell peppers, cucumbers, carrots, and hoisin sauce.
2. Spoon the mixture into lettuce leaves and wrap.

5. Chickpea and Tomato Salad

Ingredients:
- 1 can chickpeas, drained and rinsed

- 1 cup cherry tomatoes, halved
- 1/4 cup red onion, finely chopped
- 1/4 cup chopped parsley
- 2 tbsp lemon juice
- 1 tbsp olive oil
- Salt and pepper to taste

Instructions:

1. In a large bowl, combine chickpeas, cherry tomatoes, red onion, and parsley.
2. In a small bowl, whisk together lemon juice, olive oil, salt, and pepper.
3. Pour the dressing over the salad and toss to coat.

6. Cauliflower Fried Rice

Ingredients:
- 1 small head of cauliflower, grated
- 1/2 cup peas
- 1/2 cup diced carrots
- 1/4 cup diced onions
- 2 cloves garlic, minced
- 2 large eggs, beaten
- 2 tbsp soy sauce
- 1 tbsp sesame oil

Instructions:

1. In a large skillet over medium heat, heat the sesame oil.
2. Add onions, carrots, and garlic, and sauté until tender.
3. Add cauliflower rice, peas, and soy sauce, and cook until heated through.
4. Push the mixture to one side of the skillet and pour in the beaten eggs.
5. Scramble the eggs, then mix them into the cauliflower rice.

7. Mediterranean Stuffed Peppers

Ingredients:
- 4 large bell peppers, halved and seeded
- 1 cup cooked quinoa
- 1/2 cup diced tomatoes
- 1/4 cup chopped Kalamata olives
- 1/4 cup feta cheese
- 2 tbsp chopped fresh basil
- 1 tbsp olive oil
- Salt and pepper to taste

Instructions:
1. Preheat the oven to 375°F (190°C).
2. In a large bowl, combine quinoa, tomatoes, olives, feta cheese, basil, olive oil, salt, and pepper.
3. Stuff the bell peppers with the quinoa mixture.

4. Place the stuffed peppers in a baking dish and bake for 25-30 minutes.

8. Spinach and Mushroom Frittata

Ingredients:
- 6 large eggs
- 1 cup fresh spinach
- 1 cup sliced mushrooms
- 1/4 cup diced onions
- 1/4 cup grated Parmesan cheese
- 1 tbsp olive oil
- Salt and pepper to taste

Instructions:
1. Preheat the oven to 375°F (190°C).
2. In a large skillet over medium heat, heat the sesame oil.
3. Sauté onions and mushrooms until tender.
4. Add spinach and cook until wilted.
5. Whisk together eggs, Parmesan cheese, salt, and pepper in a bowl.
6. Pour the egg mixture over the vegetables in the skillet.
7. Transfer the skillet to the oven and bake for 15-20 minutes until the eggs are set.

9. Greek Salad with Grilled Shrimp

Ingredients:
- 1 cup cooked, peeled shrimp
- 2 cups mixed greens
- 1/2 cup cherry tomatoes, halved
- 1/4 cup sliced cucumbers
- 1/4 cup Kalamata olives
- 1/4 cup feta cheese
- 2 tbsp lemon juice
- 1 tbsp olive oil
- Salt and pepper to taste

Instructions:
1. In a large bowl, combine mixed greens, cherry tomatoes, cucumbers, olives, and feta cheese.
2. In a small bowl, whisk together lemon juice, olive oil, salt, and pepper.
3. Pour the dressing over the salad and toss to coat.
4. Top with grilled shrimp.

10. Spaghetti Squash with Tomato and Basil

Ingredients:
- 1 spaghetti squash, halved and seeded
- 1 cup cherry tomatoes, halved
- 1/4 cup chopped fresh basil
- 2 cloves garlic, minced
- 2 tbsp olive oil
- Salt and pepper to taste

Instructions:
1. Preheat the oven to 375°F (190°C).
2. Put the spaghetti squash halves with the cut side down on a baking sheet, then bake them for 40 minutes.
3. Using a fork, scrape the squash into strands and place in a bowl.
4. In a skillet, heat olive oil over medium heat.
5. Add garlic and tomatoes, cooking until tomatoes are softened.
6. Toss the spaghetti squash with the tomato mixture and basil.
7. Season with salt and pepper.

11. Asian Chicken Salad

Ingredients:
- 2 cups cooked, shredded chicken breast
- 2 cups shredded cabbage
- 1 cup shredded carrots
- 1/2 cup sliced almonds
- 1/4 cup chopped green onions
- 1/4 cup soy sauce
- 2 tbsp rice vinegar
- 1 tbsp sesame oil

Instructions:

1. In a large bowl, combine chicken, cabbage, carrots, almonds, and green onions.
2. In a small bowl, whisk together soy sauce, rice vinegar, and sesame oil.
3. Pour the dressing over the salad and toss to coat.

12. Turkey and Avocado Salad

Ingredients:
- 2 cups mixed greens
- 1 cup cooked turkey breast, sliced
- 1/2 avocado, sliced
- 1/4 cup dried cranberries
- 1/4 cup chopped walnuts
- 2 tbsp balsamic vinaigrette

Instructions:
1. In a large bowl, combine mixed greens, turkey, avocado, cranberries, and walnuts.
2. Drizzle with balsamic vinaigrette and toss to coat.

13. Zucchini Noodles with Pesto

Ingredients:
- 2 large zucchinis, spiralized
- 1/4 cup pesto sauce
- 1/4 cup cherry tomatoes, halved
- 1/4 cup grated Parmesan cheese

- 1 tbsp olive oil
- Salt and pepper to taste

Instructions:

1. Heat up some olive oil in a skillet over medium heat.
2. Add zucchini noodles and cook for 2-3 minutes until just tender.
3. Remove from heat and toss with pesto sauce, cherry tomatoes, and Parmesan cheese.
4. Season with salt and pepper.

14. Tuna and White Bean Salad

Ingredients:

- 1 can tuna, drained
- 1 can white beans, drained and rinsed
- 1/4 cup red onion, finely chopped
- 1/4 cup chopped parsley
- 2 tbsp lemon juice
- 1 tbsp olive oil
- Salt and pepper to taste

Instructions:

1. In a large bowl, combine tuna, white beans, red onion, and parsley.
2. In a small bowl, whisk together lemon juice, olive oil, salt, and pepper.
3. Pour the dressing over the salad and toss to coat.

15. Chicken and Veggie Stir-Fry

Ingredients:
- 1 cup cooked chicken breast, sliced
- 1 cup broccoli florets
- 1/2 cup sliced bell peppers
- 1/2 cup snap peas
- 2 cloves garlic, minced
- 2 tbsp soy sauce
- 1 tbsp sesame oil

Instructions:
1. Heat up the sesame oil in a large skillet over medium heat.
2. Add garlic and cook until fragrant.
3. Add broccoli, bell peppers, and snap peas, and cook until tender.
4. Stir in chicken and soy sauce, and cook until heated through.

16. Quinoa Stuffed Bell Peppers

Ingredients:
- 4 large bell peppers, halved and seeded
- 1 cup cooked quinoa
- 1/2 cup black beans, drained and rinsed
- 1/2 cup corn kernels

- 1/4 cup diced tomatoes
- 1/4 cup chopped cilantro
- 1 tbsp lime juice
- Salt and pepper to taste

Instructions:
1. Preheat the oven to 375°F (190°C).
2. In a large bowl, combine quinoa, black beans, corn, tomatoes, cilantro, lime juice, salt, and pepper.
3. Stuff the bell peppers with the quinoa mixture.
4. Place the stuffed peppers in a baking dish and bake for 25-30 minutes.

17. Salmon and Asparagus

Ingredients:
- 1 salmon fillet
- 1 bunch asparagus, trimmed
- 2 tbsp olive oil
- 1 tbsp lemon juice
- Salt and pepper to taste

Instructions:
1. Preheat the oven to 400°F (200°C).
2. Place salmon fillet and asparagus on a baking sheet.
3. Drizzle with olive oil and lemon juice.
4. Season with salt and pepper.

5. Bake for 15-20 minutes until salmon is cooked through and asparagus is tender.

18. Greek Chicken Bowls

Ingredients:
- 1 cup cooked quinoa
- 1 cup cooked, shredded chicken breast
- 1/2 cup cherry tomatoes, halved
- 1/4 cup diced cucumber
- 1/4 cup Kalamata olives
- 2 tbsp crumbled feta cheese
- 1 tbsp olive oil
- 1 tbsp lemon juice
- Salt and pepper to taste

Instructions:
1. In a large bowl, combine quinoa, chicken, cherry tomatoes, cucumber, olives, and feta cheese.
2. In a small bowl, whisk together olive oil, lemon juice, salt, and pepper.
3. Pour the dressing over the bowl and toss to coat.

19. Roasted Vegetable Salad

Ingredients:
- 1 cup diced sweet potatoes
- 1 cup Brussels sprouts, halved

- 1 cup diced carrots
- 2 tbsp olive oil
- Salt and pepper to taste
- 2 cups mixed greens
- 1/4 cup balsamic vinaigrette

Instructions:
1. Preheat the oven to 400°F (200°C).
2. Toss sweet potatoes, Brussels sprouts, and carrots with olive oil, salt, and pepper.
3. Spread on a baking sheet and roast for 20-25 minutes until tender.
4. In a large bowl, combine roasted vegetables and mixed greens.
5. Drizzle with balsamic vinaigrette and toss to coat.

20. Eggplant and Tomato Stew

Ingredients:
- 1 large eggplant, diced
- 1 can diced tomatoes
- 1 onion, chopped
- 2 cloves garlic, minced
- 2 tbsp olive oil
- 1 tsp oregano
- Salt and pepper to taste

Instructions:

1. Heat olive oil in a big pot on medium heat.
2. Put in onion and garlic, and sauté until they're soft and fragrant.
3. Add eggplant, tomatoes, oregano, salt, and pepper.
4. Bring to a boil, then reduce heat and simmer for 20-25 minutes until eggplant is tender.

21. Beef and Broccoli Stir-Fry

Ingredients:
- 1 cup cooked beef, sliced
- 1 cup broccoli florets
- 1/2 cup sliced bell peppers
- 2 cloves garlic, minced
- 2 tbsp soy sauce
- 1 tbsp sesame oil

Instructions:
1. Heat the sesame oil in a large skillet over medium heat.
2. Add garlic and cook until fragrant.
3. Add broccoli and bell peppers, and cook until tender.
4. Stir in beef and soy sauce, and cook until heated through.

22. Chickpea and Spinach Stew

Ingredients:

- 1 can chickpeas, drained and rinsed
- 1 can diced tomatoes
- 2 cups fresh spinach
- 1 onion, chopped
- 2 cloves garlic, minced
- 1 tbsp olive oil
- 1 tsp cumin
- Salt and pepper to taste

Instructions:
1. Heat up some olive oil in a large pot over medium heat.
2. Add the onion and garlic, and let them cook until they're nice and soft.
3. Add chickpeas, tomatoes, cumin, salt, and pepper.
4. Bring to a boil, then lower the heat and let it simmer gently for about 15-20 minutes.
5. Stir in spinach until wilted.

23. Turkey and Veggie Skewers

Ingredients:
- 1 cup cooked turkey breast, cubed
- 1 cup cherry tomatoes
- 1/2 cup diced bell peppers
- 1/2 cup diced zucchini
- 2 tbsp olive oil
- 1 tbsp lemon juice

- Salt and pepper to taste

Instructions:
1. Preheat the grill to medium-high heat.
2. Thread turkey, cherry tomatoes, bell peppers, and zucchini onto skewers.
3. Combine olive oil, lemon juice, salt, and pepper in a small bowl, and whisk them together.
4. Brush the skewers with the olive oil mixture.
5. Grill for 10-15 minutes, turning occasionally, until vegetables are tender.

24. Quinoa and Veggie Stir-Fry

Ingredients:
- 1 cup cooked quinoa
- 1 cup broccoli florets
- 1/2 cup sliced bell peppers
- 1/2 cup snap peas
- 2 cloves garlic, minced
- 2 tbsp soy sauce
- 1 tbsp sesame oil

Instructions:
1. Heat the sesame oil in a large skillet over medium heat.
2. Add garlic and cook until fragrant.

3. Add broccoli, bell peppers, and snap peas, and cook until tender.

4. Stir in quinoa and soy sauce, and cook until heated through.

25. Grilled Vegetable Wrap

Ingredients:
- 1 whole grain tortilla
- 1/2 cup grilled zucchini
- 1/2 cup grilled bell peppers
- 1/2 cup grilled eggplant
- 1/4 cup hummus
- 1/4 cup crumbled feta cheese

Instructions:
1. Spread hummus on the tortilla.
2. Layer with grilled zucchini, bell peppers, eggplant, and feta cheese.
3. Roll up the tortilla and slice in half.

26. Lentil and Veggie Stir-Fry

Ingredients:
- 1 cup cooked lentils
- 1 cup broccoli florets
- 1/2 cup sliced bell peppers
- 1/2 cup snap peas

- 2 cloves garlic, minced
- 2 tbsp soy sauce
- 1 tbsp sesame oil

Instructions:

1. Heat the sesame oil in a large skillet over medium heat.
2. Add garlic and cook until fragrant.
3. Add broccoli, bell peppers, and snap peas, and cook until tender.
4. Stir in lentils and soy sauce, and cook until heated through.

27. Avocado and Black Bean Salad

Ingredients:
- 1 can black beans, drained and rinsed
- 1 avocado, diced
- 1/2 cup cherry tomatoes, halved
- 1/4 cup red onion, finely chopped
- 1/4 cup chopped cilantro
- 2 tbsp lime juice
- 1 tbsp olive oil
- Salt and pepper to taste

Instructions:

1. In a large bowl, combine black beans, avocado, cherry tomatoes, red onion, and cilantro.

2. In a small bowl, whisk together lime juice, olive oil, salt, and pepper.
3. Pour the dressing over the salad and toss to coat.

28. Salmon and Veggie Stir-Fry

Ingredients:
- 1 cup cooked salmon, flaked
- 1 cup broccoli florets
- 1/2 cup sliced bell peppers
- 1/2 cup snap peas
- 2 cloves garlic, minced
- 2 tbsp soy sauce
- 1 tbsp sesame oil

Instructions:
1. Heat the sesame oil in a large skillet over medium heat.
2. Add garlic and cook until fragrant.
3. Add broccoli, bell peppers, and snap peas, and cook until tender.
4. Stir in salmon and soy sauce, and cook until heated through.

29. Sweet Potato and Black Bean Salad

Ingredients:
- 1 large sweet potato, diced and roasted

- 1 can black beans, drained and rinsed
- 1/2 cup diced red bell pepper
- 1/4 cup chopped cilantro
- 2 tbsp lime juice
- 1 tbsp olive oil
- Salt and pepper to taste

Instructions:
1. Preheat the oven to 400°F (200°C).
2. Toss sweet potato with olive oil, salt, and pepper.
3. Spread on a baking sheet and roast for 20-25 minutes until tender.
4. In a large bowl, combine roasted sweet potato, black beans, red bell pepper, and cilantro.
5. Drizzle with lime juice and toss to coat.

30. Tofu and Veggie Stir-Fry

Ingredients:
- 1 cup cubed tofu
- 1 cup broccoli florets
- 1/2 cup sliced bell peppers
- 1/2 cup snap peas
- 2 cloves garlic, minced
- 2 tbsp soy sauce
- 1 tbsp sesame oil

Instructions:

1. Heat the sesame oil in a large skillet over medium heat.
2. Add garlic and cook until fragrant.
3. Add tofu, broccoli, bell peppers, and snap peas, and cook until tender.
4. Stir in soy sauce and cook until heated through.

31. Chicken and Avocado Salad

Ingredients:
- 1 cup cooked, shredded chicken breast
- 1/2 avocado, diced
- 1/2 cup cherry tomatoes, halved
- 1/4 cup red onion, finely chopped
- 1/4 cup chopped cilantro
- 2 tbsp lime juice
- 1 tbsp olive oil
- Salt and pepper to taste

Instructions:
1. In a large bowl, combine chicken, avocado, cherry tomatoes, red onion, and cilantro.
2. In a small bowl, whisk together lime juice, olive oil, salt, and pepper.
3. Pour the dressing over the salad and toss to coat.

32. Shrimp and Mango Salad

Ingredients:
- 1 cup cooked, peeled shrimp
- 1/2 cup diced mango
- 1/2 cup cherry tomatoes, halved
- 1/4 cup red onion, finely chopped
- 1/4 cup chopped cilantro
- 2 tbsp lime juice
- 1 tbsp olive oil
- Salt and pepper to taste

Instructions:
1. In a large bowl, combine shrimp, mango, cherry tomatoes, red onion, and cilantro.
2. In a small bowl, whisk together lime juice, olive oil, salt, and pepper.
3. Pour the dressing over the salad and toss to coat.

33. Grilled Chicken and Veggie Bowls

Ingredients:
- 1 cup cooked quinoa
- 1 cup cooked, grilled chicken breast, sliced
- 1/2 cup grilled zucchini
- 1/2 cup grilled bell peppers
- 1/4 cup hummus
- 1/4 cup crumbled feta cheese

Instructions:

1. In a large bowl, combine quinoa, chicken, zucchini, and bell peppers.
2. Top with hummus and feta cheese.

34. Eggplant and Chickpea Stew

Ingredients:
- 1 large eggplant, diced
- 1 can chickpeas, drained and rinsed
- 1 can diced tomatoes
- 1 onion, chopped
- 2 cloves garlic, minced
- 2 tbsp olive oil
- 1 tsp cumin
- Salt and pepper to taste

Instructions:
1. Heat the olive oil in a large pot over medium heat.
2. Add onion and garlic, and cook until tender.
3. Add eggplant, chickpeas, tomatoes, cumin, salt, and pepper.
4. Bring to a boil, then reduce heat and simmer for 20-25 minutes until eggplant is tender.

35. Quinoa and Avocado Salad

Ingredients:
- 1 cup cooked quinoa

- 1/2 avocado, diced
- 1/2 cup cherry tomatoes, halved
- 1/4 cup red onion, finely chopped
- 1/4 cup chopped cilantro
- 2 tbsp lime juice
- 1 tbsp olive oil
- Salt and pepper to taste

Instructions:

1. In a large bowl, combine quinoa, avocado, cherry tomatoes, red onion, and cilantro.
2. In a small bowl, whisk together lime juice, olive oil, salt, and pepper.
3. Pour the dressing over the salad and toss to coat.

36. Tofu and Broccoli Stir-Fry

Ingredients:
- 1 cup cubed tofu
- 1 cup broccoli florets
- 1/2 cup sliced bell peppers
- 2 cloves garlic, minced
- 2 tbsp soy sauce
- 1 tbsp sesame oil

Instructions:

1. Heat the sesame oil in a large skillet over medium heat.

2. Add garlic and cook until fragrant.

3. Add tofu, broccoli, and bell peppers, and cook until tender.

4. Stir in soy sauce and cook until heated through.

37. Spinach and Chickpea Salad

Ingredients:
- 2 cups fresh spinach
- 1 can chickpeas, drained and rinsed
- 1/2 cup cherry tomatoes, halved
- 1/4 cup red onion, finely chopped
- 1/4 cup chopped parsley
- 2 tbsp lemon juice
- 1 tbsp olive oil
- Salt and pepper to taste

Instructions:
1. In a large bowl, combine spinach, chickpeas, cherry tomatoes, red onion, and parsley.

2. In a small bowl, whisk together lemon juice, olive oil, salt, and pepper.

3. Pour the dressing over the salad and toss to coat.

38. Turkey and Veggie Stir-Fry

Ingredients:
- 1 cup cooked turkey breast, sliced

- 1 cup broccoli florets
- 1/2 cup sliced bell peppers
- 2 cloves garlic, minced
- 2 tbsp soy sauce
- 1 tbsp sesame oil

Instructions:
1. Heat the sesame oil in a large skillet over medium heat.
2. Add garlic and cook until fragrant.
3. Add turkey, broccoli, and bell peppers, and cook until tender.
4. Stir in soy sauce and cook until heated through.

39. Quinoa and Black Bean Tacos

Ingredients:
- 1 cup cooked quinoa
- 1 can black beans, drained and rinsed
- 1/2 cup diced tomatoes
- 1/4 cup diced red onion
- 1/4 cup chopped cilantro
- 1 tbsp lime juice
- Whole grain tortillas

Instructions:
1. In a large bowl, combine quinoa, black beans, tomatoes, red onion, cilantro, and lime juice.

2. Spoon the mixture into tortillas and serve.

40. Lentil and Sweet Potato Stew

Ingredients:
- 1 cup cooked lentils
- 1 large sweet potato, diced
- 1 can diced tomatoes
- 1 onion, chopped
- 2 cloves garlic, minced
- 2 tbsp olive oil
- 1 tsp cumin
- Salt and pepper to taste

Instructions:
1. Heat up the olive oil in a large pot over medium heat.
2. Add onion and garlic, and cook until tender.
3. Add sweet potato, lentils, tomatoes, cumin, salt, and pepper.
4. Bring to a boil, then reduce heat and simmer for 20-25 minutes until the sweet potato is tender.

41. Zucchini Noodles with Pesto

Ingredients:
- 2 large zucchinis, spiralized
- 1/2 cup cherry tomatoes, halved
- 1/4 cup pesto sauce

- 2 tbsp grated Parmesan cheese
- Salt and pepper to taste

Instructions:
1. In a large bowl, toss zucchini noodles with pesto sauce.
2. Add cherry tomatoes and Parmesan cheese.
3. Season with salt and pepper, and serve immediately.

42. Cauliflower Fried Rice

Ingredients:
- 1 head cauliflower, grated into rice-sized pieces
- 1 cup diced carrots
- 1 cup peas
- 2 eggs, beaten
- 2 cloves garlic, minced
- 2 tbsp soy sauce
- 1 tbsp sesame oil

Instructions:
1. Heat the sesame oil in a large skillet over medium heat.
2. Add garlic and cook until fragrant.
3. Add carrots and peas, and cook until tender.
4. Stir in cauliflower rice and soy sauce, and cook until heated through.

5. Push the mixture to the side of the skillet and scramble the eggs on the other side. Mix everything together before serving.

43. Chickpea and Avocado Wrap

Ingredients:
- 1 whole grain tortilla
- 1/2 cup chickpeas, mashed
- 1/2 avocado, mashed
- 1/4 cup diced tomatoes
- 1/4 cup shredded lettuce
- 1 tbsp lemon juice
- Salt and pepper to taste

Instructions:
1. In a small bowl, combine mashed chickpeas, mashed avocado, lemon juice, salt, and pepper.
2. Spread the mixture on the tortilla.
3. Top with diced tomatoes and shredded lettuce.
4. Roll up the tortilla and slice in half.

44. Turkey and Spinach Stuffed Peppers

Ingredients:
- 4 bell peppers, halved and seeded
- 1 cup cooked ground turkey
- 2 cups fresh spinach, chopped

- 1/2 cup diced tomatoes
- 1/4 cup shredded mozzarella cheese
- Salt and pepper to taste

Instructions:
1. Preheat the oven to 375°F (190°C).
2. In a large bowl, combine ground turkey, spinach, diced tomatoes, salt, and pepper.
3. Stuff the bell peppers with the turkey mixture.
4. Place the stuffed peppers in a baking dish and top with shredded mozzarella cheese.
5. Bake for 25-30 minutes until peppers are tender and cheese is melted.

45. Shrimp and Avocado Salad

Ingredients:
- 1 cup cooked shrimp, peeled and deveined
- 1/2 avocado, diced
- 1/2 cup cherry tomatoes, halved
- 1/4 cup red onion, finely chopped
- 1/4 cup chopped cilantro
- 2 tbsp lime juice
- Salt and pepper to taste

Instructions:
1. In a large bowl, combine shrimp, avocado, cherry tomatoes, red onion, and cilantro.

2. In a small bowl, whisk together lime juice, salt, and pepper.

3. Pour the dressing over the salad and toss to coat.

46. Lentil and Kale Soup

Ingredients:
- 1 cup cooked lentils
- 2 cups chopped kale
- 1 can diced tomatoes
- 1 onion, chopped
- 2 cloves garlic, minced
- 2 tbsp olive oil
- 4 cups vegetable broth
- 1 tsp cumin
- Salt and pepper to taste

Instructions:
1. Heat up the olive oil in a big pot on medium heat.
2. Toss in the onion and garlic, and sauté until they're soft.
3. Add kale, diced tomatoes, lentils, vegetable broth, cumin, salt, and pepper.
4. Bring to a boil, then reduce heat and simmer for 20-25 minutes until kale is tender.

47. Spaghetti Squash with Marinara Sauce

Ingredients:
- 1 spaghetti squash
- 1 cup marinara sauce
- 1/4 cup grated Parmesan cheese
- 1/4 cup chopped fresh basil
- Salt and pepper to taste

Instructions:
1. Preheat the oven to 375°F (190°C).
2. Cut the spaghetti squash in half and remove seeds.
3. Place the squash halves cut-side down on a baking sheet and bake for 35-40 minutes until tender.
4. Use a fork to scrape out the strands of squash into a large bowl.
5. Toss the squash with marinara sauce, Parmesan cheese, basil, salt, and pepper.

48. Black Bean and Sweet Potato Quesadillas

Ingredients:
- 1 whole grain tortilla
- 1/2 cup mashed sweet potato
- 1/2 cup black beans, drained and rinsed
- 1/4 cup shredded cheddar cheese
- 1/4 cup diced tomatoes
- 1/4 cup chopped cilantro

- 1 tbsp olive oil

Instructions:
1. Spread mashed sweet potato on one half of the tortilla.
2. Top with black beans, cheddar cheese, diced tomatoes, and cilantro.
3. Fold the tortilla in half.
4. Heat up the olive oil in a large skillet over medium heat.
5. Cook the quesadilla until the tortilla is golden brown and the cheese is melted, about 3-4 minutes per side.

49. Grilled Salmon with Avocado Salsa

Ingredients:
- 1 salmon fillet
- 1 avocado, diced
- 1/2 cup cherry tomatoes, halved
- 1/4 cup red onion, finely chopped
- 2 tbsp lime juice
- Salt and pepper to taste
- 1 tbsp olive oil

Instructions:
1. Preheat the grill to medium-high heat.
2. Sprinkle some salt and pepper on the salmon fillet for seasoning.

3. Grill the salmon for 4-5 minutes per side until cooked through.
4. In a small bowl, combine avocado, cherry tomatoes, red onion, lime juice, salt, and pepper.
5. Serve the grilled salmon topped with avocado salsa.

50. Chickpea and Quinoa Salad

Ingredients:
- 1 cup cooked quinoa
- 1 cup cooked chickpeas
- 1/2 cup diced cucumbers
- 1/2 cup cherry tomatoes, halved
- 1/4 cup chopped parsley
- 2 tbsp lemon juice
- 1 tbsp olive oil
- Salt and pepper to taste

Instructions:
1. In a large bowl, combine quinoa, chickpeas, cucumbers, cherry tomatoes, and parsley.
2. In a small bowl, whisk together lemon juice, olive oil, salt, and pepper.
3. Pour the dressing over the salad and toss to coat.

51. Greek Yogurt Chicken Salad

Ingredients:

- 1 cup cooked, shredded chicken breast
- 1/2 cup Greek yogurt
- 1/4 cup diced celery
- 1/4 cup diced red onion
- 1/4 cup halved grapes
- 1 tbsp lemon juice
- Salt and pepper to taste

Instructions:

1. In a large bowl, combine shredded chicken, Greek yogurt, celery, red onion, grapes, lemon juice, salt, and pepper.
2. Mix well and serve chilled.

52. Roasted Beet and Goat Cheese Salad

Ingredients:
- 2 large beets, roasted and diced
- 1/4 cup crumbled goat cheese
- 2 cups mixed greens
- 1/4 cup chopped walnuts
- 2 tbsp balsamic vinaigrette

Instructions:
1. Preheat the oven to 400°F (200°C).
2. Wrap beets in foil and roast for 45-50 minutes until tender.
3. Peel and dice the roasted beets.

4. In a large bowl, combine mixed greens, diced beets, goat cheese, and walnuts.
5. Drizzle with balsamic vinaigrette and toss to coat.

53. Cauliflower Tabbouleh

Ingredients:
- 1 head cauliflower, grated into rice-sized pieces
- 1/2 cup diced cucumbers
- 1/2 cup diced tomatoes
- 1/4 cup chopped parsley
- 2 tbsp lemon juice
- 1 tbsp olive oil
- Salt and pepper to taste

Instructions:
1. In a large bowl, combine grated cauliflower, cucumbers, tomatoes, and parsley.
2. In a small bowl, whisk together lemon juice, olive oil, salt, and pepper.
3. Pour the dressing over the tabbouleh and toss to coat.

54. Baked Falafel with Tahini Sauce

Ingredients:
- 1 can chickpeas, drained and rinsed
- 1/4 cup chopped onion
- 2 cloves garlic, minced

- 2 tbsp chopped parsley
- 1 tbsp olive oil
- 1 tsp cumin
- Salt and pepper to taste
- 1/4 cup tahini
- 2 tbsp lemon juice
- Water as needed

Instructions:
1. Preheat the oven to 375°F (190°C).
2. In a food processor, combine chickpeas, onion, garlic, parsley, olive oil, cumin, salt, and pepper.
3. Process until smooth and form into small patties.
4. Place the patties on a baking sheet and bake for 20-25 minutes until golden brown.
5. In a small bowl, whisk together tahini, lemon juice, and water to make a sauce.
6. Serve the falafel with tahini sauce.

55. Spinach and Feta Stuffed Chicken Breast

Ingredients:
- 2 boneless, skinless chicken breasts
- 1 cup fresh spinach, chopped
- 1/4 cup crumbled feta cheese
- 2 cloves garlic, minced
- 1 tbsp olive oil
- Salt and pepper to taste

Instructions:
1. Preheat the oven to 375°F (190°C).
2. Cut a pocket into each chicken breast.
3. In a small bowl, combine spinach, feta cheese, garlic, salt, and pepper.
4. Stuff the mixture into the chicken breasts.
5. Heat olive oil in an oven-safe skillet over medium heat.
6. Brown the chicken on both sides, then transfer the skillet to the oven and bake for 20-25 minutes until chicken is cooked through.

56. Eggplant Rollatini

Ingredients:
- 1 large eggplant, sliced thinly lengthwise
- 1 cup ricotta cheese
- 1/4 cup grated Parmesan cheese
- 1 egg
- 1 cup marinara sauce
- 1/4 cup shredded mozzarella cheese
- Salt and pepper to taste

Instructions:
1. Preheat the oven to 375°F (190°C).
2. In a small bowl, combine ricotta cheese, Parmesan cheese, egg, salt, and pepper.

3. Spread a thin layer of marinara sauce in a baking dish.

4. Place a spoonful of the ricotta mixture on each eggplant slice and roll up.

5. Arrange the roll-ups in the baking dish, seam side down.

6. Top with remaining marinara sauce and shredded mozzarella cheese.

7. Bake for 25-30 minutes until eggplant is tender and cheese is melted.

57. Turkey and Hummus Wrap

Ingredients:
- 1 whole grain tortilla
- 1/2 cup hummus
- 1/2 cup sliced turkey breast
- 1/4 cup shredded lettuce
- 1/4 cup diced tomatoes
- 1/4 cup shredded carrots

Instructions:
1. Spread hummus on the tortilla.

2. Layer with sliced turkey, lettuce, tomatoes, and carrots.

3. Roll up the tortilla and slice in half.

58. Grilled Portobello Mushrooms

Ingredients:
- 2 large Portobello mushrooms, stems removed
- 2 tbsp balsamic vinegar
- 1 tbsp olive oil
- 2 cloves garlic, minced
- Salt and pepper to taste

Instructions:
1. Preheat the grill to medium-high heat.
2. In a small bowl, whisk together balsamic vinegar, olive oil, garlic, salt, and pepper.
3. Brush the mixture onto the Portobello mushrooms.
4. Grill the mushrooms for 4-5 minutes per side until tender.

59. Roasted Red Pepper and Lentil Soup

Ingredients:
- 1 cup cooked lentils
- 2 roasted red peppers, diced
- 1 onion, chopped
- 2 cloves garlic, minced
- 2 tbsp olive oil
- 4 cups vegetable broth
- 1 tsp smoked paprika
- Salt and pepper to taste

Instructions:

1. Heat up the olive oil in a big pot on medium heat.

2. Toss in the onion and garlic, and sauté until they're soft.

3. Add roasted red peppers, lentils, vegetable broth, smoked paprika, salt, and pepper.

4. Bring to a boil, then lower the heat and let it simmer gently for about 15-20 minutes.

60. Tuna and White Bean Salad

Ingredients:
- 1 can tuna, drained
- 1 can white beans, drained and rinsed
- 1/2 cup diced red bell pepper
- 1/4 cup chopped red onion
- 2 tbsp lemon juice
- 1 tbsp olive oil
- Salt and pepper to taste

Instructions:
1. In a large bowl, combine tuna, white beans, red bell pepper, and red onion.

2. In a small bowl, whisk together lemon juice, olive oil, salt, and pepper.

3. Pour the dressing over the salad and toss to coat.

61. Chicken and Asparagus Stir-Fry

Ingredients:
- 1 cup cooked, sliced chicken breast
- 1 cup asparagus, cut into 1-inch pieces
- 1/2 cup sliced bell peppers
- 2 cloves garlic, minced
- 2 tbsp soy sauce
- 1 tbsp sesame oil

Instructions:
1. Heat up the sesame oil in a large skillet over medium heat.
2. Add garlic and cook until fragrant.
3. Add chicken, asparagus, and bell peppers, and cook until tender.
4. Stir in soy sauce and cook until heated through.

62. Broccoli and Cheese Stuffed Potatoes

Ingredients:
- 2 medium sweet potatoes
- 1 cup cooked broccoli florets
- 1/4 cup shredded cheddar cheese
- 2 tbsp Greek yogurt
- Salt and pepper to taste

Instructions:

1. Preheat the oven to 375°F (190°C).

2. Pierce sweet potatoes with a fork and bake for 45-50 minutes until tender.

3. Cut the potatoes in half and scoop out the insides into a bowl.

4. Mash the sweet potato with Greek yogurt, salt, and pepper.

5. Stir in cooked broccoli florets and shredded cheddar cheese.

6. Spoon the mixture back into the potato skins and bake for an additional 10-15 minutes until the cheese is melted.

63. Mediterranean Chickpea Salad

Ingredients:
- 1 cup cooked chickpeas
- 1/2 cup diced cucumber
- 1/2 cup cherry tomatoes, halved
- 1/4 cup chopped red onion
- 1/4 cup crumbled feta cheese
- 2 tbsp olive oil
- 1 tbsp lemon juice
- Salt and pepper to taste

Instructions:

1. In a large bowl, combine chickpeas, cucumber, cherry tomatoes, red onion, and feta cheese.
2. Combine olive oil, lemon juice, salt, and pepper in a small bowl, and whisk until well mixed.
3. Drizzle the dressing over the salad and mix it in thoroughly.

64. Balsamic Glazed Brussels Sprouts

Ingredients:
- 2 cups Brussels sprouts, halved
- 2 tbsp balsamic vinegar
- 1 tbsp olive oil
- Salt and pepper to taste

Instructions:

1. Preheat the oven to 400°F (200°C).
2. In a large bowl, toss Brussels sprouts with balsamic vinegar, olive oil, salt, and pepper.
3. Spread the Brussels sprouts on a baking sheet and roast for 20-25 minutes until tender and caramelized.

65. Grilled Chicken and Peach Salad

Ingredients:
- 1 cup cooked, sliced chicken breast
- 1 ripe peach, sliced

- 2 cups mixed greens
- 1/4 cup crumbled goat cheese
- 2 tbsp balsamic vinaigrette

Instructions:
1. In a large bowl, combine mixed greens, sliced chicken, peach slices, and goat cheese.
2. Drizzle with balsamic vinaigrette and toss to coat.

66. Quinoa and Roasted Vegetable Bowl

Ingredients:
- 1 cup cooked quinoa
- 1 cup roasted vegetables (e.g., bell peppers, zucchini, carrots)
- 1/4 cup crumbled feta cheese
- 2 tbsp lemon tahini dressing

Instructions:
1. In a large bowl, combine cooked quinoa, roasted vegetables, and feta cheese.
2. Drizzle with lemon tahini dressing and toss to coat.

67. Turkey and Cranberry Salad

Ingredients:
- 1 cup cooked, sliced turkey breast
- 1/2 cup dried cranberries

- 1/4 cup chopped walnuts
- 2 cups mixed greens
- 2 tbsp balsamic vinaigrette

Instructions:

1. In a large bowl, combine mixed greens, turkey, cranberries, and walnuts.

2. Drizzle with balsamic vinaigrette and toss to coat.

68. Lentil and Spinach Salad

Ingredients:
- 1 cup cooked lentils
- 2 cups fresh spinach
- 1/2 cup diced cucumbers
- 1/4 cup chopped red onion
- 1/4 cup chopped parsley
- 2 tbsp lemon juice
- 1 tbsp olive oil
- Salt and pepper to taste

Instructions:

1. In a large bowl, combine lentils, spinach, cucumbers, red onion, and parsley.

2. In a small bowl, whisk together lemon juice, olive oil, salt, and pepper.

3. Pour the dressing over the salad and toss to coat.

69. Zucchini and Black Bean Enchiladas

Ingredients:
- 2 large zucchinis, sliced thinly lengthwise
- 1 cup black beans, drained and rinsed
- 1/2 cup diced tomatoes
- 1/4 cup chopped cilantro
- 1/4 cup shredded cheddar cheese
- 1 cup enchilada sauce

Instructions:
1. Preheat the oven to 375°F (190°C).
2. Spread a thin layer of enchilada sauce in a baking dish.
3. Place black beans, diced tomatoes, and cilantro on zucchini slices and roll up.
4. Arrange the roll-ups in the baking dish and top with remaining enchilada sauce and shredded cheddar cheese.
5. Bake for 20-25 minutes until zucchini is tender and cheese is melted.

70. Spinach and Artichoke Stuffed Portobello Mushrooms

Ingredients:
- 2 large Portobello mushrooms, stems removed
- 1 cup fresh spinach, chopped
- 1/2 cup canned artichoke hearts, drained and chopped

- 1/4 cup grated Parmesan cheese
- 2 cloves garlic, minced
- 1 tbsp olive oil
- Salt and pepper to taste

Instructions:
1. Preheat the oven to 375°F (190°C).
2. In a large skillet, heat olive oil over medium heat.
3. Add garlic and cook until fragrant.
4. Stir in spinach and artichoke hearts, and cook until spinach is wilted.
5. Remove from heat and stir in Parmesan cheese, salt, and pepper.
6. Stuff the Portobello mushrooms with the spinach mixture.
7. Place the mushrooms on a baking sheet and bake for 20-25 minutes until mushrooms are tender.

71. Chicken and Avocado Lettuce Wraps

Ingredients:
- 1 cup cooked, diced chicken breast
- 1/2 avocado, diced
- 1/4 cup diced tomatoes
- 1/4 cup shredded lettuce
- 2 tbsp lime juice
- Salt and pepper to taste
- Large lettuce leaves for wrapping

Instructions:

1. In a large bowl, combine chicken, avocado, tomatoes, shredded lettuce, lime juice, salt, and pepper.
2. Spoon the mixture onto large lettuce leaves and wrap.

72. Lentil and Sweet Potato Curry

Ingredients:
- 1 cup cooked lentils
- 1 large sweet potato, peeled and diced
- 1 onion, chopped
- 2 cloves garlic, minced
- 2 tbsp curry powder
- 1 can coconut milk
- 1 cup vegetable broth
- Salt and pepper to taste

Instructions:

1. Heat a large pot over medium heat.
2. Add onion and garlic, and cook until tender.
3. Stir in curry powder and cook for 1 minute.
4. Add sweet potatoes, coconut milk, vegetable broth, lentils, salt, and pepper.
5. Bring to a boil, then reduce heat and simmer for 20-25 minutes until sweet potatoes are tender.

73. Grilled Eggplant and Tomato Salad

Ingredients:
- 1 large eggplant, sliced
- 2 tomatoes, diced
- 1/4 cup chopped basil
- 2 tbsp balsamic vinegar
- 1 tbsp olive oil
- Salt and pepper to taste

Instructions:
1. Get the grill ready by preheating it to medium-high heat.
2. Coat the eggplant slices with olive oil and sprinkle them with salt and pepper.
3. Grill the eggplant for about 4-5 minutes on each side until they're tender.
4. In a large bowl, combine grilled eggplant, diced tomatoes, and basil.
5. Drizzle with balsamic vinegar and toss to coat.

74. Quinoa and Black Bean Stuffed Peppers

Ingredients:
- 4 bell peppers, halved and seeded
- 1 cup cooked quinoa
- 1 cup black beans, drained and rinsed
- 1/2 cup diced tomatoes

- 1/4 cup chopped cilantro
- 1/4 cup shredded cheddar cheese
- Salt and pepper to taste

Instructions:
1. Preheat the oven to 375°F (190°C).
2. In a large bowl, combine cooked quinoa, black beans, diced tomatoes, cilantro, salt, and pepper.
3. Stuff the bell peppers with the quinoa mixture.
4. Place the stuffed peppers in a baking dish and top with shredded cheddar cheese.
5. Bake for 25-30 minutes until peppers are tender and cheese is melted.

75. Spinach and Feta Stuffed Chicken Thighs

Ingredients:
- 4 boneless, skinless chicken thighs
- 1 cup fresh spinach, chopped
- 1/4 cup crumbled feta cheese
- 2 cloves garlic, minced
- 1 tbsp olive oil
- Salt and pepper to taste

Instructions:
1. Preheat the oven to 375°F (190°C).
2. In a small bowl, combine spinach, feta cheese, garlic, salt, and pepper.

3. Stuff the mixture under the skin of the chicken thighs.

4. Heat olive oil in an oven-safe skillet over medium heat.

5. Brown the chicken thighs on both sides, then transfer the skillet to the oven and bake for 20-25 minutes until chicken is cooked through.

76. Broccoli and Cheddar Stuffed Chicken Breast

Ingredients:
- 2 boneless, skinless chicken breasts
- 1 cup cooked broccoli florets
- 1/4 cup shredded cheddar cheese
- 2 cloves garlic, minced
- 1 tbsp olive oil
- Salt and pepper to taste

Instructions:
1. Preheat the oven to 375°F (190°C).
2. Cut a pocket into each chicken breast.
3. In a small bowl, combine cooked broccoli, shredded cheddar cheese, garlic, salt, and pepper.
4. Stuff the mixture into the chicken breasts.
5. Heat olive oil in an oven-safe skillet over medium heat.
6. Brown the chicken on both sides, then transfer the skillet to the oven and bake for 20-25 minutes until chicken is cooked through.

77. Greek Salad with Grilled Chicken

Ingredients:
- 1 cup cooked, sliced chicken breast
- 2 cups mixed greens
- 1/2 cup diced cucumbers
- 1/2 cup cherry tomatoes, halved
- 1/4 cup sliced red onion
- 1/4 cup crumbled feta cheese
- 2 tbsp olive oil
- 1 tbsp red wine vinegar
- Salt and pepper to taste

Instructions:
1. In a large bowl, combine mixed greens, chicken, cucumbers, cherry tomatoes, red onion, and feta cheese.
2. Combine olive oil, red wine vinegar, salt, and pepper in a small bowl, and whisk until well blended.
3. Drizzle the dressing over the salad and mix it in thoroughly to coat everything evenly.

78. Chickpea and Spinach Stew

Ingredients:
- 1 cup cooked chickpeas
- 2 cups fresh spinach, chopped
- 1 can diced tomatoes

- 1 onion, chopped
- 2 cloves garlic, minced
- 2 tbsp olive oil
- 4 cups vegetable broth
- 1 tsp cumin
- Salt and pepper to taste

Instructions:

1. Heat up some olive oil in a large pot over medium heat.
2. Put in the onion and garlic, and sauté them until they're soft and tender.
13. Stir in cumin and cook for 1 minute.
4. Add diced tomatoes, vegetable broth, chickpeas, spinach, salt, and pepper.
5. Bring to a boil, then reduce heat and simmer for 20-25 minutes.

79. Grilled Chicken and Vegetable Skewers

Ingredients:
- 1 cup cooked, diced chicken breast
- 1 zucchini, sliced
- 1 bell pepper, diced
- 1 red onion, diced
- 2 tbsp olive oil
- Salt and pepper to taste

Instructions:

1. Preheat the grill to medium-high heat.
2. Thread chicken, zucchini, bell pepper, and red onion onto skewers.
3. Coat with olive oil and sprinkle with salt and pepper.
4. Grill for 4-5 minutes per side until vegetables are tender and chicken is heated through.

80. Spinach and Mushroom Stuffed Peppers

Ingredients:
- 4 bell peppers, halved and seeded
- 1 cup fresh spinach, chopped
- 1 cup sliced mushrooms
- 1/4 cup shredded mozzarella cheese
- 2 cloves garlic, minced
- 1 tbsp olive oil
- Salt and pepper to taste

Instructions:
1. Preheat the oven to 375°F (190°C).
2. In a large skillet, heat olive oil over medium heat.
3. Add garlic and cook until fragrant.
4. Stir in spinach and mushrooms, and cook until spinach is wilted and mushrooms are tender.
5. Season with salt and pepper.
6. Stuff the bell peppers with the spinach and mushroom mixture.

7. Place the stuffed peppers in a baking dish and top with shredded mozzarella cheese.
8. Bake for 20-25 minutes until peppers are tender and cheese is melted.

81. Turkey and Spinach Meatballs

Ingredients:
- 1 cup ground turkey
- 1 cup fresh spinach, chopped
- 1/4 cup grated Parmesan cheese
- 1 egg
- 2 cloves garlic, minced
- 1 tbsp olive oil
- Salt and pepper to taste

Instructions:
1. Preheat the oven to 375°F (190°C).
2. In a large bowl, combine ground turkey, spinach, Parmesan cheese, egg, garlic, salt, and pepper.
3. Form the mixture into small meatballs and place on a baking sheet.
4. Drizzle with olive oil and bake for 20-25 minutes until cooked through.

82. Lentil and Cauliflower Curry

Ingredients:
- 1 cup cooked lentils
- 1 head cauliflower, cut into florets
- 1 onion, chopped
- 2 cloves garlic, minced
- 2 tbsp curry powder
- 1 can coconut milk
- 1 cup vegetable broth
- Salt and pepper to taste

Instructions:
1. Heat a large pot over medium heat.
2. Put in the onion and garlic, and sauté until they're soft.
3. Mix in the curry powder and cook for about a minute.
4. Add cauliflower, coconut milk, vegetable broth, lentils, salt, and pepper.
5. Bring to a boil, then reduce heat and simmer for 20-25 minutes until the cauliflower is tender.

83. Grilled Chicken and Pineapple Skewers

Ingredients:
- 1 cup cooked, diced chicken breast
- 1 cup pineapple chunks
- 1 bell pepper, diced
- 1 red onion, diced

- 2 tbsp olive oil
- Salt and pepper to taste

Instructions:
1. Preheat the grill to medium-high heat.
2. Thread chicken, pineapple, bell pepper, and red onion onto skewers.
3. Brush with olive oil and season with salt and pepper.
4. Grill for 4-5 minutes per side until vegetables are tender and chicken is heated through.

84. Spinach and Ricotta Stuffed Shells

Ingredients:
- 1 cup ricotta cheese
- 1 cup fresh spinach, chopped
- 1/4 cup grated Parmesan cheese
- 1 egg
- 1 cup marinara sauce
- 1/4 cup shredded mozzarella cheese
- Salt and pepper to taste
- Large pasta shells

Instructions:
1. Preheat the oven to 375°F (190°C).
2. In a large pot, cook pasta shells according to package instructions.

3. In a large bowl, combine ricotta cheese, spinach, Parmesan cheese, egg, salt, and pepper.

4. Spread a thin layer of marinara sauce in a baking dish.

5. Stuff the pasta shells with the ricotta mixture and arrange in the baking dish.

6. Top with remaining marinara sauce and shredded mozzarella cheese.

7. Bake for 25-30 minutes until cheese is melted and bubbly.

85. Turkey and Avocado Salad

Ingredients:
- 1 cup cooked, sliced turkey breast
- 1/2 avocado, diced
- 2 cups mixed greens
- 1/4 cup cherry tomatoes, halved
- 2 tbsp lemon juice
- 1 tbsp olive oil
- Salt and pepper to taste

Instructions:
1. In a large bowl, combine mixed greens, turkey, avocado, and cherry tomatoes.

2. In a small bowl, whisk together lemon juice, olive oil, salt, and pepper.

3. Pour the dressing over the salad and toss to coat.

86. Baked Falafel

Ingredients:
- 1 cup cooked chickpeas
- 1/4 cup chopped parsley
- 2 cloves garlic, minced
- 1/4 cup chopped onion
- 1 tbsp olive oil
- 1 tsp ground cumin
- Salt and pepper to taste
- 1 tbsp flour

Instructions:
1. Preheat the oven to 375°F (190°C).
2. In a food processor, combine chickpeas, parsley, garlic, onion, olive oil, cumin, salt, pepper, and flour.
3. Pulse until well combined but still slightly chunky.
4. Form the mixture into small patties and place on a baking sheet.
5. Bake for 20-25 minutes until golden brown, flipping halfway through.

87. Grilled Eggplant and Zucchini Salad

Ingredients:
- 1 large eggplant, sliced
- 2 zucchinis, sliced
- 1/4 cup chopped basil

- 2 tbsp balsamic vinegar
- 1 tbsp olive oil
- Salt and pepper to taste

Instructions:
1. Preheat the grill to medium-high heat.
2. Brush eggplant and zucchini slices with olive oil and season with salt and pepper.
3. Grill vegetables for 4-5 minutes per side until tender.
4. In a large bowl, combine grilled eggplant, zucchini, and basil.
5. Drizzle with balsamic vinegar and toss to coat.

88. Turkey and Spinach Stuffed Mushrooms

Ingredients:
- 4 large Portobello mushrooms, stems removed
- 1 cup cooked ground turkey
- 1 cup fresh spinach, chopped
- 1/4 cup grated Parmesan cheese
- 2 cloves garlic, minced
- 1 tbsp olive oil
- Salt and pepper to taste

Instructions:
1. Preheat the oven to 375°F (190°C).
2. In a large skillet, heat olive oil over medium heat.
3. Add garlic and cook until fragrant.

4. Stir in ground turkey and spinach, and cook until spinach is wilted.

5. Season with salt and pepper.

6. Stuff the mushrooms with the turkey and spinach mixture.

7. Place the stuffed mushrooms on a baking sheet and top with grated Parmesan cheese.

8. Bake for 20-25 minutes until mushrooms are tender.

89. Lentil and Butternut Squash Stew

Ingredients:
- 1 cup cooked lentils
- 1 cup diced butternut squash
- 1 onion, chopped
- 2 cloves garlic, minced
- 2 tbsp olive oil
- 4 cups vegetable broth
- 1 tsp ground cumin
- Salt and pepper to taste

Instructions:
1. Heat olive oil in a large pot over medium heat.
2. Add onion and garlic, and cook until tender.
3. Stir in cumin and cook for 1 minute.
4. Add butternut squash, vegetable broth, lentils, salt, and pepper.

5. Bring to a boil, then reduce heat and simmer for 20-25 minutes until butternut squash is tender.

90. Grilled Chicken and Avocado Salad

Ingredients:
- 1 cup cooked, sliced chicken breast
- 1/2 avocado, diced
- 2 cups mixed greens
- 1/4 cup cherry tomatoes, halved
- 2 tbsp lemon juice
- 1 tbsp olive oil
- Salt and pepper to taste

Instructions:
1. In a large bowl, combine mixed greens, chicken, avocado, and cherry tomatoes.
2. In a small bowl, whisk together lemon juice, olive oil, salt, and pepper.
3. Pour the dressing over the salad and toss to coat.

91. Balsamic Glazed Carrots

Ingredients:
- 2 cups baby carrots
- 2 tbsp balsamic vinegar
- 1 tbsp olive oil
- 1 tbsp honey

- Salt and pepper to taste

Instructions:
1. Preheat the oven to 400°F (200°C).
2. In a large bowl, toss carrots with balsamic vinegar, olive oil, honey, salt, and pepper.
3. Spread the carrots on a baking sheet and roast for 20-25 minutes until tender and caramelized.

92. Turkey and Sweet Potato Skillet

Ingredients:
- 1 cup cooked, diced turkey breast
- 1 large sweet potato, peeled and diced
- 1 onion, chopped
- 2 cloves garlic, minced
- 2 tbsp olive oil
- Salt and pepper to taste

Instructions:
1. Heat olive oil in a large skillet over medium heat.
2. Add onion and garlic, and cook until tender.
3. Stir in diced sweet potato, and cook until tender.
4. Add turkey, salt, and pepper, and cook until heated through.

93. Spinach and Goat Cheese Stuffed Mushrooms

Ingredients:
- 4 large Portobello mushrooms, stems removed
- 1 cup fresh spinach, chopped
- 1/4 cup crumbled goat cheese
- 2 cloves garlic, minced
- 1 tbsp olive oil
- Salt and pepper to taste

Instructions:
1. Preheat the oven to 375°F (190°C).
2. In a large skillet, heat olive oil over medium heat.
3. Add garlic and cook until fragrant.
4. Stir in spinach and cook until wilted.
5. Remove from heat and stir in goat cheese, salt, and pepper.
6. Stuff the mushrooms with the spinach mixture.
7. Place the stuffed mushrooms on a baking sheet and bake for 20-25 minutes until mushrooms are tender.

94. Lentil and Vegetable Stir-Fry

Ingredients:
- 1 cup cooked lentils
- 1 cup mixed vegetables (e.g., bell peppers, broccoli, snap peas)
- 2 cloves garlic, minced
- 2 tbsp soy sauce
- 1 tbsp sesame oil

Instructions:

1. Heat up the sesame oil in a large skillet over medium heat.

2. Toss in the onion and garlic, and sauté until they're soft.

3. Add mixed vegetables and cook until tender.

4. Stir in lentils and soy sauce, and cook until heated through.

95. Grilled Chicken and Mango Salad

Ingredients:
- 1 cup cooked, sliced chicken breast
- 1 ripe mango, diced
- 2 cups mixed greens
- 1/4 cup chopped red onion
- 2 tbsp lime juice
- 1 tbsp olive oil
- Salt and pepper to taste

Instructions:

1. In a large bowl, combine mixed greens, chicken, mango, and red onion.

2. In a small bowl, whisk together lime juice, olive oil, salt, and pepper.

3. Pour the dressing over the salad and toss to coat.

96. Zucchini and Feta Fritters

Ingredients:
- 2 zucchinis, grated
- 1/4 cup crumbled feta cheese
- 1 egg
- 2 tbsp flour
- 2 cloves garlic, minced
- 1 tbsp olive oil
- Salt and pepper to taste

Instructions:
1. In a large bowl, combine grated zucchini, feta cheese, egg, flour, garlic, salt, and pepper.
2. Heat up the olive oil in a large skillet over medium heat.
3. Drop spoonfuls of the zucchini mixture into the skillet and flatten slightly.
4. Cook for 3-4 minutes per side until golden brown and crispy.

97. Spinach and Mushroom Quiche

Ingredients:
- 1 cup fresh spinach, chopped
- 1 cup sliced mushrooms
- 1/2 cup shredded cheddar cheese
- 4 eggs

- 1 cup milk
- 1 pre-made pie crust
- Salt and pepper to taste

Instructions:
1. Preheat the oven to 375°F (190°C).
2. In a large skillet, cook spinach and mushrooms until tender.
3. In a large bowl, whisk together eggs, milk, salt, and pepper.
4. Stir in cooked spinach, mushrooms, and cheddar cheese.
5. Pour the mixture into the pie crust.
6. Bake for 30-35 minutes until the quiche is set and the crust is golden brown.

98. Baked Tofu and Vegetable Stir-Fry

Ingredients:
- 1 block firm tofu, cubed
- 1 cup mixed vegetables (e.g., bell peppers, broccoli, snap peas)
- 2 cloves garlic, minced
- 2 tbsp soy sauce
- 1 tbsp sesame oil

Instructions:
1. Preheat the oven to 400°F (200°C).

2. Spread tofu cubes on a baking sheet and bake for 20-25 minutes until golden and crispy.

3. Heat up the sesame oil in a large skillet over medium heat.

4. Add garlic and cook until fragrant.

5. Add mixed vegetables and cook until tender.

6. Stir in baked tofu and soy sauce, and cook until heated through.

99. Grilled Chicken and Strawberry Salad

Ingredients:
- 1 cup cooked, sliced chicken breast
- 1 cup sliced strawberries
- 2 cups mixed greens
- 1/4 cup crumbled feta cheese
- 2 tbsp balsamic vinegar
- 1 tbsp olive oil
- Salt and pepper to taste

Instructions:
1. In a large bowl, combine mixed greens, chicken, strawberries, and feta cheese.

2. Mix balsamic vinegar, olive oil, salt, and pepper in a small bowl.

3.Then, drizzle it over the salad and give it a good toss to make sure everything's coated."

100. Lentil and Sweet Potato Burgers

Ingredients:
- 1 cup cooked lentils
- 1 cup mashed sweet potatoes
- 1/4 cup grated carrots
- 1/4 cup chopped onion
- 2 cloves garlic, minced
- 1 tbsp olive oil
- 1/4 cup flour
- Salt and pepper to taste

Instructions:
1. In a large bowl, combine cooked lentils, mashed sweet potatoes, grated carrots, onion, garlic, flour, salt, and pepper.
2. Form the mixture into patties.
3. Heat up the olive oil in a large skillet over medium heat.
4. Cook patties for 3-4 minutes per side until golden brown and crispy.

These nutrient-dense low glycemic lunch recipes offer a variety of flavors and ingredients to keep your meals interesting and nutritious. Enjoy experimenting with these dishes and discovering your favorites.

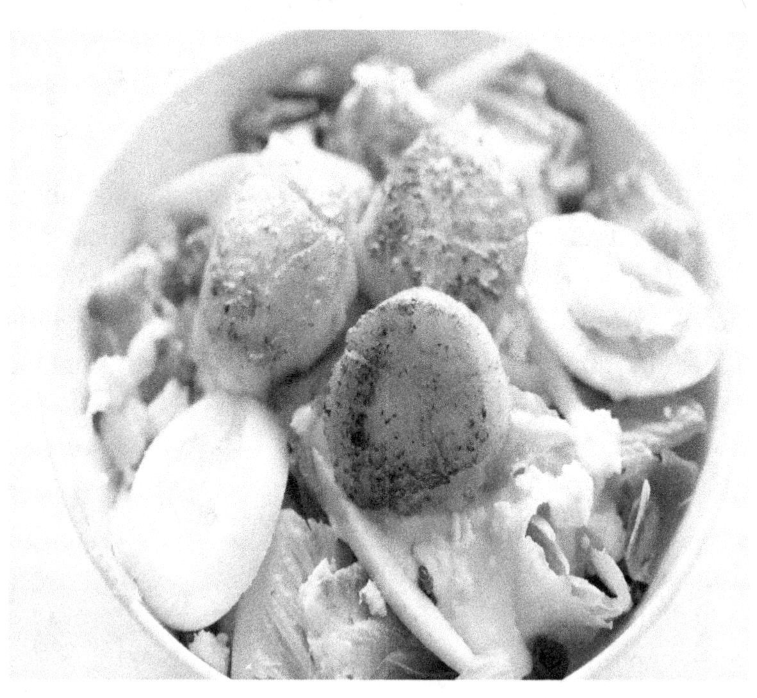

Chapter 5: Healthy and Nutritious Low Glycemic Dinner Feast Recipes

Creating a low glycemic dinner feast is all about selecting the right ingredients and combining them in a way that satisfies both your taste buds and nutritional needs. Here are delicious and nutrient-dense low glycemic dinner recipes that are sure to delight you and your family.

1. Lemon Herb Grilled Salmon

Ingredients:
- 4 salmon fillets
- 1/4 cup olive oil
- 2 lemons, juiced
- 2 cloves garlic, minced
- 1 tbsp chopped fresh dill
- 1 tbsp chopped fresh parsley
- Salt and pepper to taste

Instructions:
1. In a small bowl, whisk together olive oil, lemon juice, garlic, dill, parsley, salt, and pepper.

2. Place salmon fillets in a shallow dish and pour the marinade over them. Let marinate for 30 minutes.
3. Preheat the grill to medium-high heat.
4. Grill salmon for 4-5 minutes per side until fully cooked.
5. Serve with a side of steamed vegetables.

2. Quinoa Stuffed Bell Peppers

Ingredients:
- 4 large bell peppers, halved and seeded
- 1 cup cooked quinoa
- 1/2 cup black beans, drained and rinsed
- 1/2 cup corn kernels
- 1/4 cup diced tomatoes
- 1/4 cup chopped cilantro
- 1 tsp cumin
- Salt and pepper to taste

Instructions:
1. Preheat the oven to 375°F (190°C).
2. In a large bowl, combine quinoa, black beans, corn, tomatoes, cilantro, cumin, salt, and pepper.
3. Stuff the bell peppers with the quinoa mixture.
4. Place the stuffed peppers in a baking dish and bake for 25-30 minutes until peppers are tender.

3. Balsamic Glazed Chicken and Vegetables

Ingredients:
- 4 boneless, skinless chicken breasts
- 1/4 cup balsamic vinegar
- 2 tbsp olive oil
- 2 cloves garlic, minced
- 1 cup cherry tomatoes, halved
- 1 zucchini, sliced
- 1 red onion, sliced
- Salt and pepper to taste

Instructions:
1. Preheat the oven to 400°F (200°C).
2. In a small bowl, whisk together balsamic vinegar, olive oil, garlic, salt, and pepper.
3. Place chicken breasts in a baking dish and arrange tomatoes, zucchini, and onion around the chicken.
4. Pour the balsamic mixture over the chicken and vegetables.
5. Bake for 25-30 minutes until chicken is cooked through and vegetables are tender.

4. Spaghetti Squash with Pesto and Shrimp

Ingredients:
- 1 large spaghetti squash
- 1/4 cup basil pesto
- 1 lb shrimp, peeled and deveined

- 2 cloves garlic, minced
- 2 tbsp olive oil
- Salt and pepper to taste

Instructions:
1. Preheat the oven to 400°F (200°C).
2. Cut the spaghetti squash in half lengthwise and scoop out the seeds.
3. Place the squash halves cut-side down on a baking sheet and bake for 40-45 minutes until tender.
4. Heat some olive oil in a big skillet pan on medium heat.
5. Add garlic and cook until fragrant.
6. Add shrimp and cook until pink and opaque, about 3-4 minutes.
7. Using a fork, scrape the flesh of the squash into strands and transfer to a large bowl.
8. Toss the squash with pesto, shrimp, salt, and pepper.

5. Chicken and Vegetable Stir-Fry

Ingredients:
- 1 lb boneless, skinless chicken breast, sliced
- 1 cup broccoli florets
- 1 red bell pepper, sliced
- 1 yellow bell pepper, sliced
- 1 carrot, julienned
- 2 cloves garlic, minced

- 2 tbsp soy sauce
- 1 tbsp sesame oil
- 1 tbsp olive oil

Instructions:
1. Heat some olive oil in a big skillet pan on medium heat.
2. Add chicken and cook until browned and cooked through, about 5-7 minutes. Remove and set aside.
3. In the same skillet, add sesame oil and garlic. Cook until fragrant.
4. Add broccoli, bell peppers, and carrot. Stir-fry until vegetables are tender, about 5-7 minutes.
5. Return chicken to the skillet and add soy sauce. Toss to combine and heat through.

6. Turkey Meatballs with Zucchini Noodles

Ingredients:
- 1 lb ground turkey
- 1/4 cup grated Parmesan cheese
- 1/4 cup chopped fresh parsley
- 1 egg
- 2 cloves garlic, minced
- 1 tbsp olive oil
- 4 large zucchinis, spiralized into noodles
- 1 cup marinara sauce
- Salt and pepper to taste

Instructions:
1. Preheat the oven to 375°F (190°C).
2. In a large bowl, combine ground turkey, Parmesan cheese, parsley, egg, garlic, salt, and pepper.
3. Form mixture into meatballs and place on a baking sheet. Bake for 20-25 minutes until cooked through.
4. Heat some olive oil in a big skillet pan on medium heat.
5. Add zucchini noodles and cook until just tender, about 2-3 minutes.
6. Serve meatballs over zucchini noodles with marinara sauce.

7. Cauliflower Fried Rice

Ingredients:
- 1 head cauliflower, grated or processed into rice-sized pieces
- 1 cup mixed vegetables (carrots, peas, corn)
- 2 eggs, beaten
- 2 cloves garlic, minced
- 2 tbsp soy sauce
- 1 tbsp sesame oil
- 2 green onions, sliced

Instructions:

1. Heat some olive oil in a big skillet pan on medium heat.

2. Add garlic and cook until fragrant.

3. Stir in cauliflower rice and mixed vegetables. Cook until tender, about 5-7 minutes.

4. Push the cauliflower mixture to one side of the skillet and add the beaten eggs to the other side. Scramble the eggs until cooked through.

5. Stir in soy sauce and green onions. Mix everything together and serve.

8. Baked Cod with Lemon and Dill

Ingredients:
- 4 cod fillets
- 1/4 cup olive oil
- 2 lemons, juiced and zested
- 2 cloves garlic, minced
- 1 tbsp chopped fresh dill
- Salt and pepper to taste

Instructions:

1. Preheat the oven to 375°F (190°C).

2. In a small bowl, whisk together olive oil, lemon juice, lemon zest, garlic, dill, salt, and pepper.

3. Place cod fillets in a baking dish and pour the lemon mixture over them.

4. Bake for 20-25 minutes until the cod is flaky and cooked through.

9. Eggplant Lasagna

Ingredients:
- 2 large eggplants, sliced lengthwise
- 1 cup ricotta cheese
- 1 cup shredded mozzarella cheese
- 1 egg
- 2 cups marinara sauce
- 1/4 cup grated Parmesan cheese
- Salt and pepper to taste

Instructions:
1. Preheat the oven to 375°F (190°C).
2. Sprinkle eggplant slices with salt and let sit for 15 minutes to draw out moisture. Pat dry.
3. In a large bowl, mix ricotta cheese, egg, salt, and pepper.
4. Spread a thin layer of marinara sauce in a baking dish.
5. Layer with eggplant slices, ricotta mixture, and mozzarella cheese. Repeat layers.
6. Top with remaining marinara sauce and Parmesan cheese.
7. Bake for 30-35 minutes until cheese is melted and bubbly.

10. Beef and Broccoli Stir-Fry

Ingredients:
- 1 lb flank steak, thinly sliced
- 1 cup broccoli florets
- 1 red bell pepper, sliced
- 2 cloves garlic, minced
- 2 tbsp soy sauce
- 1 tbsp oyster sauce
- 1 tbsp sesame oil
- 1 tbsp olive oil

Instructions:
1. Heat some olive oil in a big frying pan on medium heat.
2. Add steak and cook until browned, about 4-5 minutes. Remove and set aside.
3. In the same skillet, add sesame oil and garlic. Cook until fragrant.
4. Add broccoli and bell pepper. Stir-fry until tender, about 5-7 minutes.
5. Return steak to the skillet and add soy sauce and oyster sauce. Toss to combine and heat through.

11. Chicken and Spinach Stuffed Portobello Mushrooms

Ingredients:

- 4 large Portobello mushrooms, stems removed
- 1 cup cooked, shredded chicken breast
- 1 cup fresh spinach, chopped
- 1/4 cup grated Parmesan cheese
- 2 cloves garlic, minced
- 1 tbsp olive oil
- Salt and pepper to taste

Instructions:
1. Preheat the oven to 375°F (190°C).
2. In a large skillet, heat olive oil over medium heat.
3. Add garlic and cook until fragrant.
4. Stir in chicken and spinach, and cook until spinach is wilted.
5. Season with salt and pepper.
6. Stuff the mushrooms with the chicken mixture.
7. Place the stuffed mushrooms on a baking sheet and top with Parmesan cheese.
8. Bake for 20-25 minutes until mushrooms are tender.

12. Lentil and Vegetable Soup

Ingredients:
- 1 cup lentils, rinsed
- 1 onion, chopped
- 2 carrots, diced
- 2 celery stalks, diced
- 2 cloves garlic, minced

- 4 cups vegetable broth
- 1 tsp cumin
- 1 tsp thyme
- Salt and pepper to taste

Instructions:
1. In a large pot, heat up the olive oil over medium heat.
2. Add onion, carrots, celery, and garlic. Cook until tender.
3. Stir in cumin and thyme, and cook for 1 minute.
4. Add lentils and vegetable broth. Bring to a boil.
5. Reduce heat and simmer for 20-25 minutes until lentils are tender.
6. Season with salt and pepper.

13. Grilled Chicken with Mango Salsa

Ingredients:
- 4 boneless, skinless chicken breasts
- 1 ripe mango, diced
- 1/4 cup red onion, finely chopped
- 1/4 cup chopped cilantro
- 1 lime, juiced
- 1 tbsp olive oil
- Salt and pepper to taste

Instructions:
1. Preheat the grill to medium-high heat.

2. In a small bowl, combine mango, red onion, cilantro, lime juice, salt, and pepper.
3. Brush chicken breasts with olive oil and season with salt and pepper.
4. Grill chicken for 6-7 minutes per side until fully cooked.
5. Serve chicken topped with mango salsa.

14. Zucchini and Ground Turkey Skillet

Ingredients:
- 1 lb ground turkey
- 2 zucchinis, diced
- 1 red bell pepper, diced
- 1 onion, chopped
- 2 cloves garlic, minced
- 1 tbsp olive oil
- 1 tsp paprika
- Salt and pepper to taste

Instructions:
1. Get a big pot and heat up some olive oil on medium heat.
2. Toss in the onion and garlic and cook them until they're nice and soft.
3. Stir in ground turkey, breaking it apart with a spoon, and cook until browned.

4. Add zucchini, bell pepper, paprika, salt, and pepper. Cook until vegetables are tender, about 7-8 minutes.

15. Baked Lemon Herb Chicken Thighs

Ingredients:
- 4 chicken thighs, bone-in and skin-on
- 1/4 cup olive oil
- 2 lemons, juiced and zested
- 2 cloves garlic, minced
- 1 tbsp chopped fresh rosemary
- 1 tbsp chopped fresh thyme
- Salt and pepper to taste

Instructions:
1. Preheat the oven to 375°F (190°C).
2. In a small bowl, whisk together olive oil, lemon juice, lemon zest, garlic, rosemary, thyme, salt, and pepper.
3. Place chicken thighs in a baking dish and pour the lemon herb mixture over them.
4. Bake for 35-40 minutes until chicken is cooked through and skin is crispy.

16. Cauliflower and Chickpea Curry

Ingredients:
- 1 head cauliflower, cut into florets
- 1 cup cooked chickpeas

- 1 onion, chopped
- 2 cloves garlic, minced
- 1 tbsp curry powder
- 1 tsp turmeric
- 1 tsp cumin
- 1 cup coconut milk
- 1 cup vegetable broth
- Salt and pepper to taste

Instructions:

1. Get a big pot and heat up some olive oil on medium heat.
2. Toss in the onion and garlic and cook them until they're nice and soft.
3. Stir in curry powder, turmeric, and cumin, and cook for 1 minute.
4. Add cauliflower, chickpeas, coconut milk, and vegetable broth. Bring to a boil.
5. Reduce heat and simmer for 20-25 minutes until the cauliflower is tender.
6. Season with salt and pepper.

17. Spaghetti Squash with Meatballs

Ingredients:
- 1 large spaghetti squash
- 1 lb ground beef
- 1/4 cup grated Parmesan cheese

- 1 egg
- 2 cloves garlic, minced
- 1 cup marinara sauce
- Salt and pepper to taste

Instructions:
1. Preheat the oven to 400°F (200°C).
2. Cut the spaghetti squash in half lengthwise and scoop out the seeds.
3. Place the squash halves cut-side down on a baking sheet and bake for 40-45 minutes until tender.
4. In a large bowl, combine ground beef, Parmesan cheese, egg, garlic, salt, and pepper. Form mixture into meatballs.
5. Heat olive oil in a large skillet over medium heat. Cook meatballs until browned on all sides and cooked through, about 8-10 minutes.
6. In a small pot, heat marinara sauce until warm.
7. Using a fork, scrape the flesh of the squash into strands and transfer to a large bowl.
8. Serve meatballs over spaghetti squash with marinara sauce.

18. Shrimp and Avocado Salad

Ingredients:
- 1 lb shrimp, peeled and deveined
- 1/2 avocado, diced

- 2 cups mixed greens
- 1/4 cup cherry tomatoes, halved
- 2 tbsp lime juice
- 1 tbsp olive oil
- Salt and pepper to taste

Instructions:
1. In a large bowl, combine mixed greens, shrimp, avocado, and cherry tomatoes.
2. In a small bowl, whisk together lime juice, olive oil, salt, and pepper.
3. Pour the dressing over the salad and toss to coat.

19. Chicken and Broccoli Alfredo

Ingredients:
- 1 lb boneless, skinless chicken breast, sliced
- 1 cup broccoli florets
- 2 cloves garlic, minced
- 1 cup heavy cream
- 1/2 cup grated Parmesan cheese
- 1 tbsp olive oil
- Salt and pepper to taste

Instructions:
1. Heat up the olive oil in a large skillet over medium heat.

2. Add chicken and cook until browned and cooked through, about 5-7 minutes.
3. Add garlic and cook until fragrant.
4. Stir in heavy cream and bring to a simmer.
5. Add broccoli and cook until tender, about 5 minutes.
6. Stir in Parmesan cheese, salt, and pepper.

20. Baked Lemon Garlic Tilapia

Ingredients:
- 4 tilapia fillets
- 1/4 cup olive oil
- 2 lemons, juiced and zested
- 2 cloves garlic, minced
- 1 tbsp chopped fresh parsley
- Salt and pepper to taste

Instructions:
1. Preheat the oven to 375°F (190°C).
2. In a small bowl, whisk together olive oil, lemon juice, lemon zest, garlic, parsley, salt, and pepper.
3. Place tilapia fillets in a baking dish and pour the lemon garlic mixture over them.
4. Bake for 20-25 minutes until tilapia is flaky and cooked through.

21. Beef and Vegetable Skewers

Ingredients:
- 1 lb beef sirloin, cut into cubes
- 1 red bell pepper, cut into chunks
- 1 yellow bell pepper, cut into chunks
- 1 zucchini, sliced
- 1 red onion, cut into chunks
- 1/4 cup olive oil
- 2 tbsp soy sauce
- 2 cloves garlic, minced
- Salt and pepper to taste

Instructions:
1. Preheat the grill to medium-high heat.
2. In a small bowl, whisk together olive oil, soy sauce, garlic, salt, and pepper.
3. Thread beef, bell peppers, zucchini, and onion onto skewers.
4. Brush with the olive oil mixture.
5. Grill for 4-5 minutes per side until beef is cooked to desired doneness and vegetables are tender.

22. Chicken Fajita Bowls

Ingredients:
- 1 lb boneless, skinless chicken breast, sliced
- 1 red bell pepper, sliced

- 1 green bell pepper, sliced
- 1 onion, sliced
- 2 cloves garlic, minced
- 1 tbsp olive oil
- 1 tsp chili powder
- 1 tsp cumin
- 2 cups cooked quinoa
- 1/4 cup chopped cilantro
- 1 lime, juiced
- Salt and pepper to taste

Instructions:

1. Heat up the olive oil in a large skillet over medium heat.
2. Add chicken, garlic, chili powder, and cumin. Cook until chicken is browned and cooked through, about 5-7 minutes.
3. Add bell peppers and onion. Cook until tender, about 5 minutes.
4. In a large bowl, combine quinoa, cilantro, lime juice, salt, and pepper.
5. Serve chicken and vegetables over quinoa.

23. Baked Parmesan Crusted Chicken

Ingredients:
- 4 boneless, skinless chicken breasts
- 1/2 cup grated Parmesan cheese

- 1/4 cup almond flour
- 2 cloves garlic, minced
- 1 tsp paprika
- 1 tbsp olive oil
- Salt and pepper to taste

Instructions:
1. Preheat the oven to 375°F (190°C).
2. In a small bowl, combine Parmesan cheese, almond flour, garlic, paprika, salt, and pepper.
3. Brush chicken breasts with olive oil.
4. Press the Parmesan mixture onto the chicken breasts.
5. Place chicken in a baking dish and bake for 25-30 minutes until golden and cooked through.

24. Shrimp and Vegetable Stir-Fry

Ingredients:
- 1 lb shrimp, peeled and deveined
- 1 cup broccoli florets
- 1 red bell pepper, sliced
- 1 carrot, julienned
- 2 cloves garlic, minced
- 2 tbsp soy sauce
- 1 tbsp sesame oil
- 1 tbsp olive oil

Instructions:

1. Heat up the olive oil in a large skillet over medium-high heat.

2. Add shrimp and cook until pink and opaque, about 3-4 minutes. Remove and set aside.

3. In the same skillet, add sesame oil and garlic. Cook until fragrant.

4. Add broccoli, bell pepper, and carrot. Stir-fry until tender, about 5-7 minutes.

5. Return shrimp to the skillet and add soy sauce. Toss to combine and heat through.

25. Lemon Garlic Chicken Thighs

Ingredients:
- 4 chicken thighs, bone-in and skin-on
- 1/4 cup olive oil
- 2 lemons, juiced and zested
- 2 cloves garlic, minced
- 1 tbsp chopped fresh rosemary
- Salt and pepper to taste

Instructions:

1. Preheat the oven to 375°F (190°C).

2. In a small bowl, whisk together olive oil, lemon juice, lemon zest, garlic, rosemary, salt, and pepper.

3. Place chicken thighs in a baking dish and pour the lemon garlic mixture over them.

4. Bake for 35-40 minutes until chicken is cooked through and skin is crispy.

26. Spaghetti Squash Primavera

Ingredients:
- 1 large spaghetti squash
- 1 zucchini, diced
- 1 yellow squash, diced
- 1 red bell pepper, diced
- 1 cup cherry tomatoes, halved
- 2 cloves garlic, minced
- 1 tbsp olive oil
- 1/4 cup grated Parmesan cheese
- Salt and pepper to taste

Instructions:
1. Preheat the oven to 400°F (200°C).
2. Cut the spaghetti squash in half lengthwise and scoop out the seeds.
3. Place the squash halves cut-side down on a baking sheet and bake for 40-45 minutes until tender.
4. In a large skillet, heat up the olive oil over medium heat.
5. Add garlic and cook until fragrant.
6. Add zucchini, yellow squash, bell pepper, and cherry tomatoes. Cook until tender, about 5-7 minutes.

7. Using a fork, scrape the flesh of the squash into strands and transfer to a large bowl.

8. Toss the squash with the vegetable mixture, Parmesan cheese, salt, and pepper.

27. Beef and Vegetable Kabobs

Ingredients:
- 1 lb beef sirloin, cut into cubes
- 1 red bell pepper, cut into chunks
- 1 yellow bell pepper, cut into chunks
- 1 zucchini, sliced
- 1 red onion, cut into chunks
- 1/4 cup olive oil
- 2 tbsp soy sauce
- 2 cloves garlic, minced
- Salt and pepper to taste

Instructions:
1. Preheat the grill to medium-high heat.
2. In a small bowl, whisk together olive oil, soy sauce, garlic, salt, and pepper.
3. Thread beef, bell peppers, zucchini, and onion onto skewers.
4. Brush with the olive oil mixture.
5. Grill for 4-5 minutes per side until beef is cooked to desired doneness and vegetables are tender.

28. Chicken and Asparagus Stir-Fry

Ingredients:
- 1 lb boneless, skinless chicken breast, sliced
- 1 bunch asparagus, cut into 2-inch pieces
- 1 red bell pepper, sliced
- 2 cloves garlic, minced
- 2 tbsp soy sauce
- 1 tbsp sesame oil
- 1 tbsp olive oil

Instructions:
1. Heat up the olive oil in a large skillet over medium-high heat.
2. Add chicken and cook until browned and cooked through, about 5-7 minutes. Remove and set aside.
3. In the same skillet, add sesame oil and garlic. Cook until fragrant.
4. Add asparagus and bell pepper. Stir-fry until tender, about 5-7 minutes.
5. Return chicken to the skillet and add soy sauce. Toss to combine and heat through.

29. Lemon Herb Grilled Shrimp

Ingredients:
- 1 lb shrimp, peeled and deveined
- 1/4 cup olive oil

- 2 lemons, juiced and zested
- 2 cloves garlic, minced
- 1 tbsp chopped fresh parsley
- Salt and pepper to taste

Instructions:
1. In a small bowl, whisk together olive oil, lemon juice, lemon zest, garlic, parsley, salt, and pepper.
2. Place shrimp in a shallow dish and pour the marinade over them. Let marinate for 30 minutes.
3. Preheat the grill to medium-high heat.
4. Grill shrimp for 2-3 minutes per side until pink and opaque.

30. Stuffed Bell Peppers with Quinoa and Black Beans

Ingredients:
- 4 large bell peppers, halved and seeded
- 1 cup cooked quinoa
- 1/2 cup black beans, drained and rinsed
- 1/2 cup corn kernels
- 1/4 cup diced tomatoes
- 1/4 cup chopped cilantro
- 1 tsp cumin
- Salt and pepper to taste

Instructions:

1. Preheat the oven to 375°F (190°C).

2. In a large bowl, combine quinoa, black beans, corn, tomatoes, cilantro, cumin, salt, and pepper.

3. Stuff the bell peppers with the quinoa mixture.

4. Place the stuffed peppers in a baking dish and bake for 25-30 minutes until peppers are tender.

31. Grilled Chicken and Vegetable Skewers

Ingredients:
- 1 lb boneless, skinless chicken breast, cut into cubes
- 1 red bell pepper, cut into chunks
- 1 yellow bell pepper, cut into chunks
- 1 zucchini, sliced
- 1 red onion, cut into chunks
- 1/4 cup olive oil
- 2 cloves garlic, minced
- Salt and pepper to taste

Instructions:
1. Preheat the grill to medium-high heat.

2. In a small bowl, whisk together olive oil, garlic, salt, and pepper.

3. Thread chicken, bell peppers, zucchini, and onion onto skewers.

4. Brush with the olive oil mixture.

5. Grill for 4-5 minutes per side until chicken is cooked through and vegetables are tender.

32. Baked Lemon Herb Cod

Ingredients:
- 4 cod fillets
- 1/4 cup olive oil
- 2 lemons, juiced and zested
- 2 cloves garlic, minced
- 1 tbsp chopped fresh dill
- Salt and pepper to taste

Instructions:
1. Preheat the oven to 375°F (190°C).
2. In a small bowl, whisk together olive oil, lemon juice, lemon zest, garlic, dill, salt, and pepper.
3. Place cod fillets in a baking dish and pour the lemon herb mixture over them.
4. Bake for 20-25 minutes until the cod is flaky and cooked through.

33. Chicken and Cauliflower Rice Stir-Fry

Ingredients:
- 1 lb boneless, skinless chicken breast, sliced
- 1 head cauliflower, grated or processed into rice-sized pieces
- 1 cup mixed vegetables (carrots, peas, corn)
- 2 cloves garlic, minced

- 2 tbsp soy sauce
- 1 tbsp sesame oil
- 1 tbsp olive oil

Instructions:
1. Heat up olive oil in a large skillet over medium heat.
2. Add chicken and cook until browned and cooked through, about 5-7 minutes. Remove and set aside.
3. In the same skillet, add sesame oil and garlic. Cook until fragrant.
4. Add cauliflower rice and mixed vegetables. Cook until tender, about 5-7 minutes.
5. Return chicken to the skillet and add soy sauce. Toss to combine and heat through.

34. Shrimp and Avocado Salad

Ingredients:
- 1 lb shrimp, peeled and deveined
- 1/2 avocado, diced
- 2 cups mixed greens
- 1/4 cup cherry tomatoes, halved
- 2 tbsp lime juice
- 1 tbsp olive oil
- Salt and pepper to taste

Instructions:

1. In a large bowl, combine mixed greens, shrimp, avocado, and cherry tomatoes.
2. In a small bowl, whisk together lime juice, olive oil, salt, and pepper.
3. Pour the dressing over the salad and toss to coat.

35. Lemon Herb Baked Chicken Thighs

Ingredients:
- 4 chicken thighs, bone-in and skin-on
- 1/4 cup olive oil
- 2 lemons, juiced and zested
- 2 cloves garlic, minced
- 1 tbsp chopped fresh rosemary
- Salt and pepper to taste

Instructions:
1. Preheat the oven to 375°F (190°C).
2. In a small bowl, whisk together olive oil, lemon juice, lemon zest, garlic, rosemary, salt, and pepper.
3. Place chicken thighs in a baking dish and pour the lemon herb mixture over them.
4. Bake for 35-40 minutes until chicken is cooked through and skin is crispy.

36. Spaghetti Squash with Pesto and Chicken

Ingredients:

- 1 large spaghetti squash
- 1 lb boneless, skinless chicken breast, sliced
- 1/2 cup pesto
- 1/4 cup grated Parmesan cheese
- 2 cloves garlic, minced
- 1 tbsp olive oil
- Salt and pepper to taste

Instructions:

1. Preheat the oven to 400°F (200°C).
2. Cut the spaghetti squash in half lengthwise and scoop out the seeds.
3. Place the squash halves cut-side down on a baking sheet and bake for 40-45 minutes until tender.
4. In a large skillet, heat up the olive oil over medium heat.
5. Add chicken and cook until browned and cooked through, about 5-7 minutes.
6. Using a fork, scrape the flesh of the squash into strands and transfer to a large bowl.
7. Toss the squash with the chicken, pesto, Parmesan cheese, salt, and pepper.

37. Beef and Broccoli Stir-Fry

Ingredients:

- 1 lb beef sirloin, sliced thinly
- 2 cups broccoli florets

- 2 cloves garlic, minced
- 2 tbsp soy sauce
- 1 tbsp sesame oil
- 1 tbsp olive oil

Instructions:

1. Heat up the olive oil in a large skillet over medium-high heat.

2. Add beef and cook until browned and cooked through, about 5-7 minutes. Remove and set aside.

3. In the same skillet, add sesame oil and garlic. Cook until fragrant.

4. Add broccoli and stir-fry until tender, about 5-7 minutes.

5. Return beef to the skillet and add soy sauce. Toss to combine and heat through.

38. Lemon Garlic Shrimp Pasta

Ingredients:
- 1 lb shrimp, peeled and deveined
- 8 oz whole wheat pasta
- 2 cloves garlic, minced
- 1/4 cup olive oil
- 1 lemon, juiced and zested
- 1 tbsp chopped fresh parsley
- Salt and pepper to taste

Instructions:

1. Cook pasta according to package instructions.
2. In a large skillet, heat olive oil over medium heat.
3. Add garlic and cook until fragrant.
4. Add shrimp and cook until pink and opaque, about 3-4 minutes.
5. Stir in lemon juice, lemon zest, salt, and pepper.
6. Toss the cooked pasta with the shrimp mixture and sprinkle with parsley.

39. Chicken and Vegetable Stir-Fry

Ingredients:
- 1 lb boneless, skinless chicken breast, sliced
- 1 cup broccoli florets
- 1 red bell pepper, sliced
- 1 carrot, julienned
- 2 cloves garlic, minced
- 2 tbsp soy sauce
- 1 tbsp sesame oil
- 1 tbsp olive oil

Instructions:

1. Heat up olive oil in a large skillet over medium-high heat.
2. Add chicken and cook until browned and cooked through, about 5-7 minutes. Remove and set aside.

3. In the same skillet, add sesame oil and garlic. Cook until fragrant.

4. Add broccoli, bell pepper, and carrot. Stir-fry until tender, about 5-7 minutes.

5. Return chicken to the skillet and add soy sauce. Toss to combine and heat through.

40. Grilled Lemon Herb Chicken

Ingredients:
- 4 boneless, skinless chicken breasts
- 1/4 cup olive oil
- 2 lemons, juiced and zested
- 2 cloves garlic, minced
- 1 tbsp chopped fresh parsley
- Salt and pepper to taste

Instructions:
1. In a small bowl, whisk together olive oil, lemon juice, lemon zest, garlic, parsley, salt, and pepper.

2. Place chicken breasts in a shallow dish and pour the marinade over them. Let marinate for 30 minutes.

3. Preheat the grill to medium-high heat.

4. Grill chicken for 6-7 minutes per side until fully cooked.

41. Zucchini Noodles with Pesto and Shrimp

Ingredients:
- 1 lb shrimp, peeled and deveined
- 3 zucchinis, spiralized into noodles
- 1/2 cup pesto
- 2 cloves garlic, minced
- 1 tbsp olive oil
- Salt and pepper to taste

Instructions:
1. In a large skillet, heat up olive oil over medium heat.
2. Add garlic and cook until fragrant.
3. Add shrimp and cook until pink and opaque, about 3-4 minutes.
4. Stir in zucchini noodles and cook until tender, about 2-3 minutes.
5. Toss with pesto, salt, and pepper.

42. Turkey and Sweet Potato Skillet

Ingredients:
- 1 lb ground turkey
- 2 sweet potatoes, diced
- 1 red bell pepper, diced
- 1 onion, chopped
- 2 cloves garlic, minced
- olive oil
- 1 tsp paprika
- Salt and pepper to taste

Instructions:

1. Begin by heating the olive oil in a sizable skillet over medium heat.

2. Toss the onion and garlic, and saute until they reach a soft, tender texture.

2. Add onion and garlic, and cook until tender.

3. Stir in ground turkey, breaking it apart with a spoon, and cook until browned.

4. Add sweet potatoes, bell pepper, paprika, salt, and pepper. Cook until vegetables are tender, about 10-12 minutes.

43. Baked Lemon Herb Salmon

Ingredients:
- 4 salmon fillets
- 1/4 cup olive oil
- 2 lemons, juiced and zested
- 2 cloves garlic, minced
- 1 tbsp chopped fresh dill
- Salt and pepper to taste

Instructions:

1. Preheat the oven to 375°F (190°C).

2. In a small bowl, whisk together olive oil, lemon juice, lemon zest, garlic, dill, salt, and pepper.

3. Place salmon fillets in a baking dish and pour the lemon herb mixture over them.

4. Bake for 20-25 minutes until salmon is flaky and cooked through.

44. Chicken and Zucchini Noodles Stir-Fry

Ingredients:
- 1 lb boneless, skinless chicken breast, sliced
- 3 zucchinis, spiralized into noodles
- 1 red bell pepper, sliced
- 2 cloves garlic, minced
- 2 tbsp soy sauce
- 1 tbsp sesame oil
- 1 tbsp olive oil

Instructions:
1. Heat up olive oil in a large skillet over medium-high heat.

2. Add chicken and cook until browned and cooked through, about 5-7 minutes. Remove and set aside.

3. In the same skillet, add sesame oil and garlic. Cook until fragrant.

4. Add zucchini noodles and bell pepper. Stir-fry until tender, about 5-7 minutes.

5. Return chicken to the skillet and add soy sauce. Toss to combine and heat through.

45. Spaghetti Squash with Meat Sauce

Ingredients:
- 1 large spaghetti squash
- 1 lb ground beef
- 1 onion, chopped
- 2 cloves garlic, minced
- 1 cup marinara sauce
- 1/4 cup grated Parmesan cheese
- Salt and pepper to taste

Instructions:
1. Preheat the oven to 400°F (200°C).
2. Cut the spaghetti squash in half lengthwise and scoop out the seeds.
3. Place the squash halves cut-side down on a baking sheet and bake for 40-45 minutes until tender.
4. In a large skillet, heat up olive oil over medium heat.
5. Add onion and garlic, and cook until tender.
6. Stir in ground beef, breaking it apart with a spoon, and cook until browned.
7. Add marinara sauce, salt, and pepper. Cook until heated through.
8. Using a fork, scrape the flesh of the squash into strands and transfer to a large bowl.

9. Toss the squash with the meat sauce and Parmesan cheese.

46. Lemon Herb Chicken Breasts

Ingredients:
- 4 boneless, skinless chicken breasts
- 1/4 cup olive oil
- 2 lemons, juiced and zested
- 2 cloves garlic, minced
- 1 tbsp chopped fresh rosemary
- Salt and pepper to taste

Instructions:
1. In a small bowl, whisk together olive oil, lemon juice, lemon zest, garlic, rosemary, salt, and pepper.
2. Place chicken breasts in a shallow dish and pour the marinade over them. Let marinate for 30 minutes.
3. Preheat the grill to medium-high heat.
4. Grill chicken for 6-7 minutes per side until fully cooked.

47. Shrimp and Asparagus Stir-Fry

Ingredients:
- 1 lb shrimp, peeled and deveined
- 1 bunch asparagus, cut into 2-inch pieces
- 2 cloves garlic, minced

- 2 tbsp soy sauce
- 1 tbsp sesame oil
- 1 tbsp olive oil

Instructions:

1. Heat up olive oil in a large skillet over medium-high heat.

2. Add shrimp and cook until pink and opaque, about 3-4 minutes. Remove and set aside.

3. In the same skillet, add sesame oil and garlic. Cook until fragrant.

4. Add asparagus and stir-fry until tender, about 5-7 minutes.

5. Return shrimp to the skillet and add soy sauce. Toss to combine and heat through.

48. Chicken and Sweet Potato Stir-Fry

Ingredients:
- 1 lb boneless, skinless chicken breast, sliced
- 2 sweet potatoes, diced
- 1 red bell pepper, sliced
- 2 cloves garlic, minced
- 2 tbsp soy sauce
- 1 tbsp sesame oil
- 1 tbsp olive oil

Instructions:

1. Heat up olive oil in a large skillet over medium-high heat.

2. Add chicken and cook until browned and cooked through, about 5-7 minutes. Remove and set aside.

3. In the same skillet, add sesame oil and garlic. Cook until fragrant.

4. Add sweet potatoes and bell pepper. Stir-fry until tender, about 10-12 minutes.

5. Return chicken to the skillet and add soy sauce. Toss to combine and heat through.

49. Lemon Herb Shrimp Skewers

Ingredients:
- 1 lb shrimp, peeled and deveined
- 1/4 cup olive oil
- 2 lemons, juiced and zested
- 2 cloves garlic, minced
- 1 tbsp chopped fresh parsley
- Salt and pepper to taste

Instructions:
1. In a small bowl, whisk together olive oil, lemon juice, lemon zest, garlic, parsley, salt, and pepper.

2. Thread shrimp on skewers and pour the marinade over them. Let marinate for 30 minutes.

3. Preheat the grill to medium-high heat.

4. Grill shrimp for 2-3 minutes per side until pink and opaque.

50. Beef and Cauliflower Rice Stir-Fry

Ingredients:
- 1 lb beef sirloin, sliced thinly
- 1 head cauliflower, grated or processed into rice-sized pieces
- 1 cup mixed vegetables (carrots, peas, corn)
- 2 cloves garlic, minced
- 2 tbsp soy sauce
- 1 tbsp sesame oil
- 1 tbsp olive oil

Instructions:
1. Heat up olive oil in a large skillet over medium-high heat.
2. Add beef and cook until browned and cooked through, about 5-7 minutes. Remove and set aside.
3. In the same skillet, add sesame oil and garlic. Cook until fragrant.
4. Add cauliflower rice and mixed vegetables. Cook until tender, about 5-7 minutes.
5. Return beef to the skillet and add soy sauce. Toss to combine and heat through.

51. Balsamic Glazed Chicken with Brussels Sprouts

Ingredients:
- 4 boneless, skinless chicken breasts
- 2 cups Brussels sprouts, halved
- 1/4 cup balsamic vinegar
- 2 tbsp honey
- 2 cloves garlic, minced
- 2 tbsp olive oil
- Salt and pepper to taste

Instructions:
1. Preheat the oven to 400°F (200°C).
2. In a small bowl, whisk together balsamic vinegar, honey, garlic, salt, and pepper.
3. Heat up olive oil in a large oven-safe skillet over medium-high heat.
4. Add chicken breasts and cook until browned on both sides, about 3-4 minutes per side. Remove from the skillet and set aside.
5. Add Brussels sprouts to the skillet and cook until browned, about 5 minutes.
6. Return chicken to the skillet, pour balsamic mixture over chicken and Brussels sprouts.
7. Transfer skillet to the oven and bake for 15-20 minutes until chicken is cooked through.

52. Moroccan Spiced Chickpea Stew

Ingredients:
- 1 can chickpeas, drained and rinsed
- 1 onion, chopped
- 2 cloves garlic, minced
- 1 carrot, diced
- 1 red bell pepper, diced
- 1 zucchini, diced
- 1 can diced tomatoes
- 1 cup vegetable broth
- 1 tsp ground cumin
- 1 tsp ground coriander
- 1 tsp ground cinnamon
- 1 tbsp olive oil
- Salt and pepper to taste

Instructions:
1. Begin by heating the olive oil in a sizable skillet over medium heat.
2. Add the onion and garlic, cook until they are soft and tender.
3. Stir in carrot, bell pepper, and zucchini. Cook for 5-7 minutes until vegetables are tender.
4. Add chickpeas, diced tomatoes, vegetable broth, cumin, coriander, cinnamon, salt, and pepper. Bring to a boil.
5. Reduce heat and simmer for 20 minutes until flavors meld.

53. Lemon Garlic Butter Salmon

Ingredients:
- 4 salmon fillets
- 1/4 cup butter, melted
- 2 cloves garlic, minced
- 1 lemon, juiced and zested
- 1 tbsp chopped fresh parsley
- Salt and pepper to taste

Instructions:
1. Preheat the oven to 375°F (190°C).
2. In a small bowl, mix melted butter, garlic, lemon juice, lemon zest, parsley, salt, and pepper.
3. Place salmon fillets in a baking dish and pour the lemon garlic butter over them.
4. Bake for 15-20 minutes until salmon is cooked through and flaky.

54. Turkey and Spinach Stuffed Peppers

Ingredients:
- 4 large bell peppers, halved and seeded
- 1 lb ground turkey
- 2 cups fresh spinach, chopped
- 1 onion, chopped
- 2 cloves garlic, minced
- 1 cup cooked quinoa

- 1/2 cup tomato sauce
- 1 tbsp olive oil
- Salt and pepper to taste

Instructions:
1. Preheat the oven to 375°F (190°C).
2. Begin by heating the olive oil in a sizable skillet over medium heat.
3. Add the onion and garlic, cook until they are soft and tender.
4. Stir in ground turkey and cook until browned.
5. Add spinach, quinoa, tomato sauce, salt, and pepper. Cook until spinach is wilted.
6. Stuff bell peppers with the turkey mixture and place in a baking dish.
7. Cover with foil and bake for 30 minutes.

55. Thai Coconut Curry Chicken

Ingredients:
- 1 lb boneless, skinless chicken breast, sliced
- 1 onion, chopped
- 2 cloves garlic, minced
- 1 red bell pepper, sliced
- 1 cup broccoli florets
- 1 can coconut milk
- 2 tbsp red curry paste
- 1 tbsp fish sauce

- 1 tbsp olive oil
- Fresh basil leaves for garnish
- Salt and pepper to taste

Instructions:
1. Begin by heating the olive oil in a sizable skillet over medium heat.
2. Add the onion and garlic, cook until they are soft and tender.
3. Stir in chicken and cook until browned.
4. Add bell pepper, broccoli, coconut milk, red curry paste, fish sauce, salt, and pepper. Bring to a simmer.
5. Cook for 10-15 minutes until chicken is cooked through and vegetables are tender.
6. Garnish with fresh basil leaves before serving.

56. Herb-Crusted Pork Tenderloin

Ingredients:
- 1 pork tenderloin
- 2 cloves garlic, minced
- 1 tbsp chopped fresh rosemary
- 1 tbsp chopped fresh thyme
- 1 tbsp olive oil
- Salt and pepper to taste

Instructions:
1. Preheat the oven to 400°F (200°C).

2. In a small bowl, mix garlic, rosemary, thyme, olive oil, salt, and pepper.
3. Rub the herb mixture all over the pork tenderloin.
4. Place tenderloin on a baking sheet and bake for 25-30 minutes until internal temperature reaches 145°F (63°C).
5. Let rest for 5 minutes before slicing.

57. Greek Stuffed Chicken Breasts

Ingredients:
- 4 boneless, skinless chicken breasts
- 1/2 cup crumbled feta cheese
- 1/2 cup chopped spinach
- 1/4 cup sun-dried tomatoes, chopped
- 1 tbsp olive oil
- 1 tbsp lemon juice
- Salt and pepper to taste

Instructions:
1. Preheat the oven to 375°F (190°C).
2. In a small bowl, mix feta cheese, spinach, sun-dried tomatoes, salt, and pepper.
3. Cut a pocket into each chicken breast and stuff with the feta mixture.
4. Place chicken breasts in a baking dish and drizzle with olive oil and lemon juice.
5. Bake for 25-30 minutes until chicken is cooked through.

58. Quinoa and Black Bean Stuffed Acorn Squash

Ingredients:
- 2 acorn squash, halved and seeded
- 1 cup cooked quinoa
- 1/2 cup black beans, drained and rinsed
- 1/4 cup corn kernels
- 1/4 cup diced tomatoes
- 1/4 cup chopped cilantro
- 1 tsp cumin
- 1 tbsp olive oil
- Salt and pepper to taste

Instructions:
1. Preheat the oven to 375°F (190°C).
2. Place acorn squash halves cut-side down on a baking sheet and bake for 30-35 minutes until tender.
3. In a large bowl, combine quinoa, black beans, corn, tomatoes, cilantro, cumin, olive oil, salt, and pepper.
4. Stuff the acorn squash halves with the quinoa mixture.
5. Return to the oven and bake for 10-15 minutes until heated through.

59. Mediterranean Baked Cod

Ingredients:
- 4 cod fillets

- 1 can diced tomatoes
- 1/4 cup kalamata olives, pitted and halved
- 1/4 cup chopped fresh parsley
- 2 cloves garlic, minced
- 1 tbsp olive oil
- 1 tbsp lemon juice
- Salt and pepper to taste

Instructions:

1. Preheat the oven to 375°F (190°C).
2. In a small bowl, mix diced tomatoes, olives, parsley, garlic, olive oil, lemon juice, salt, and pepper.
3. Place cod fillets in a baking dish and pour the tomato mixture over them.
4. Bake for 20-25 minutes until the cod is flaky and cooked through.

60. Sesame Ginger Tofu Stir-Fry

Ingredients:
- 1 block firm tofu, drained and cubed
- 1 cup broccoli florets
- 1 red bell pepper, sliced
- 1 carrot, julienned
- 2 cloves garlic, minced
- 2 tbsp soy sauce
- 1 tbsp sesame oil
- 1 tbsp olive oil

- 1 tsp grated fresh ginger
- Sesame seeds for garnish
- Salt and pepper to taste

Instructions:
1. Heat up olive oil in a large skillet over medium-high heat.
2. Add tofu and cook until golden brown on all sides. Remove and set aside.
3. In the same skillet, add sesame oil, garlic, and ginger. Cook until fragrant.
4. Add broccoli, bell pepper, and carrot. Stir-fry until tender, about 5-7 minutes.
5. Return tofu to the skillet and add soy sauce. Toss to combine and heat through.
6. Garnish with sesame seeds before serving.

Chapter 6:Nutrient-Dense Low Glycemic Desserts and Snacks

Adopting a low glycemic diet doesn't mean giving up on delicious desserts and satisfying snacks. In fact, there are numerous ways to create nutrient-dense, low glycemic treats that satisfy your sweet tooth and snack cravings without causing a rapid spike in blood sugar. Here are 50 detailed recipes for low glycemic desserts and 50 for snacks that are both nutritious and delightful.

Low Glycemic Desserts

1. Almond Flour Chocolate Chip Cookies

Ingredients:
- 2 cups almond flour
- 1/2 cup dark chocolate chips
- 1/4 cup coconut oil, melted
- 1/4 cup honey
- 1 tsp vanilla extract
- 1/2 tsp baking soda
- 1/4 tsp salt

Instructions:

1. Preheat the oven to 350°F (175°C).

2. In a bowl, mix almond flour, baking soda, and salt.

3. In another bowl, combine melted coconut oil, honey, and vanilla extract.

4. Mix the wet ingredients into the dry ingredients until well combined.

5. Fold in the dark chocolate chips.

6. Use a spoon to place dollops of dough onto a baking sheet lined with parchment paper.

7. Bake in the oven for 10 to 12 minutes or until the cookies turn golden brown.

2. Greek Yogurt and Berry Parfait

Ingredients:

- 2 cups Greek yogurt
- 1 cup mixed berries (blueberries, strawberries, raspberries)
- 1/4 cup chopped nuts (almonds, walnuts)
- 2 tbsp chia seeds
- 2 tbsp honey

Instructions:

1. Layer Greek yogurt, mixed berries, and honey in serving glasses.

2. Sprinkle it with chia seeds and chopped nuts.

3. Serve immediately or refrigerate for later.

3. Avocado Chocolate Mousse

Ingredients:
- 2 ripe avocados
- 1/4 cup unsweetened cocoa powder
- 1/4 cup honey
- 1/4 cup almond milk
- 1 tsp vanilla extract
- Pinch of salt

Instructions:
1. Blend avocados, cocoa powder, honey, almond milk, vanilla extract, and salt until smooth.
2. Divide into serving dishes and chill for at least 30 minutes before serving.

4. Coconut Flour Brownies

Ingredients:
- 1/2 cup coconut flour
- 1/2 cup cocoa powder
- 1/2 cup coconut oil, melted
- 1/4 cup honey
- 4 eggs
- 1 tsp vanilla extract
- 1/2 tsp baking soda
- 1/4 tsp salt

Instructions:

1. Preheat the oven to 350°F (175°C).
2. In a bowl, mix coconut flour, cocoa powder, baking soda, and salt.
3. In another bowl, whisk eggs, melted coconut oil, honey, and vanilla extract.
4. Mix the wet and dry ingredients together thoroughly.
5. Transfer the batter into a baking pan that has been lightly greased.
6. Bake for 20-25 minutes until a toothpick inserted comes out clean.

5. Chia Seed Pudding

Ingredients:
- 1 cup almond milk
- 1/4 cup chia seeds
- 2 tbsp honey
- 1 tsp vanilla extract
- Fresh berries for topping

Instructions:

1. In a bowl, mix almond milk, chia seeds, honey, and vanilla extract.
2. Cover and refrigerate overnight or for at least 4 hours.
3. Serve topped with fresh berries.

6. Baked Apples with Cinnamon

Ingredients:
- 4 large apples, cored
- 1/4 cup chopped nuts (walnuts, pecans)
- 2 tbsp honey
- 1 tsp ground cinnamon
- 1/4 cup raisins

Instructions:
1. Preheat the oven to 375°F (190°C).
2. Place cored apples in a baking dish.
3. In a small bowl, mix chopped nuts, honey, ground cinnamon, and raisins.
4. Stuff each apple with the nut mixture.
5. Bake for 25-30 minutes until the apples are tender.

7. Banana Oat Cookies

Ingredients:
- 2 ripe bananas, mashed
- 1 cup rolled oats
- 1/4 cup dark chocolate chips
- 1/4 cup chopped nuts (optional)
- 1 tsp vanilla extract
- 1/2 tsp ground cinnamon

Instructions:
1. Preheat the oven to 350°F (175°C).
2. In a bowl, mix mashed bananas, rolled oats, dark chocolate chips, chopped nuts (if using), vanilla extract, and ground cinnamon.
3. Drop spoonfuls of dough onto a baking sheet lined with parchment paper.
4. Bake for 12-15 minutes until golden brown.

8. Lemon Blueberry Muffins

Ingredients:
- 1 cup almond flour
- 1/2 cup coconut flour
- 1/4 cup honey
- 3 eggs
- 1/4 cup coconut oil, melted
- 1 cup blueberries
- 1 tsp vanilla extract
- 1 tsp baking powder
- 1/4 tsp salt
- Zest of 1 lemon

Instructions:
1. Preheat the oven to 350°F (175°C).
2. In a bowl, mix almond flour, coconut flour, baking powder, and salt.

3. In another bowl, whisk eggs, honey, melted coconut oil, vanilla extract, and lemon zest.
4. Mix the wet and dry ingredients until it is well mixed.
5. Fold in blueberries.
6. Divide batter into a muffin tin lined with paper liners.
7. Bake for 20-25 minutes until a toothpick inserted comes out clean.

9. Chocolate Avocado Truffles

Ingredients:
- 2 ripe avocados
- 1/4 cup unsweetened cocoa powder
- 1/4 cup honey
- 1 tsp vanilla extract
- 1/4 cup shredded coconut (optional for rolling)

Instructions:
1. Blend avocados, cocoa powder, honey, and vanilla extract until smooth.
2. Chill the mixture for 1 hour.
3. Scoop and roll into small balls, then roll in shredded coconut if desired.
4. Store in the refrigerator.

10. Strawberry Coconut Bars

Ingredients:

- 2 cups shredded coconut
- 1/2 cup coconut oil, melted
- 1/4 cup honey
- 1 cup fresh strawberries, chopped

Instructions:

1. In a bowl, mix shredded coconut, melted coconut oil, and honey.
2. Press the mixture into a baking dish lined with parchment paper.
3. Spread chopped strawberries over the coconut mixture.
4. Refrigerate for at least 2 hours until set.
5. Cut into bars before serving.

11. Pumpkin Pie Chia Pudding

Ingredients:
- 1 cup almond milk
- 1/2 cup pumpkin puree
- 1/4 cup chia seeds
- 2 tbsp honey
- 1 tsp pumpkin pie spice
- 1 tsp vanilla extract

Instructions:

1. In a bowl, mix almond milk, pumpkin puree, chia seeds, honey, pumpkin pie spice, and vanilla extract.

2. Cover and refrigerate overnight or for at least 4 hours.
3. Serve chilled.

12. Raspberry Almond Crumble

Ingredients:
- 2 cups raspberries
- 1 cup almond flour
- 1/4 cup chopped almonds
- 2 tbsp honey
- 2 tbsp coconut oil, melted
- 1 tsp vanilla extract
- Pinch of salt

Instructions:
1. Preheat the oven to 350°F (175°C).
2. Place raspberries in a baking dish.
3. In a bowl, mix almond flour, chopped almonds, honey, melted coconut oil, vanilla extract, and salt.
4. Sprinkle the crumble mixture over the raspberries.
5. Bake for 20-25 minutes until golden brown.

13. Dark Chocolate Almond Bark

Ingredients:
- 1 cup dark chocolate chips
- 1/2 cup almonds, chopped
- 1/4 cup dried cranberries

Instructions:
1. Melt dark chocolate chips in a microwave-safe bowl, stirring every 30 seconds until smooth.
2. Stir in chopped almonds and dried cranberries.
3. Spread the mixture evenly over a baking sheet that has been lined with parchment paper.
4. Refrigerate until set, then break into pieces.

14. Coconut Macaroons

Ingredients:
- 2 cups shredded coconut
- 1/4 cup coconut flour
- 1/4 cup honey
- 1/4 cup coconut oil, melted
- 1 tsp vanilla extract
- 2 egg whites

Instructions:
1. Preheat the oven to 350°F (175°C).
2. In a bowl, mix shredded coconut, coconut flour, honey, melted coconut oil, and vanilla extract.
3. In a separate bowl, whip the egg whites until they form stiff peaks.
4. Carefully fold the whipped egg whites into the coconut mixture.

5. Drop spoonfuls of the mixture onto a baking sheet lined with parchment paper.
6. Bake for 15-20 minutes until golden brown.

15. Apple Cinnamon Energy Bites

Ingredients:
- 1 cup rolled oats
- 1/4 cup almond butter
- 1/4 cup honey
- 1/2 cup dried apples, chopped
- 1 tsp ground cinnamon
- 1 tsp vanilla extract

Instructions:
1. In a large bowl, mix rolled oats, almond butter, honey, dried apples, ground cinnamon, and vanilla extract.
2. Form the mixture into small balls.
3. Refrigerate for at least 30 minutes before serving.

16. Blueberry Chia Jam

Ingredients:
- 2 cups fresh blueberries
- 2 tbsp chia seeds
- 1-2 tbsp honey (optional)
- 1 tsp lemon juice

Instructions:
1. In a small saucepan, cook blueberries over medium heat until they begin to break down.
2. Mash the blueberries with a fork and stir in chia seeds, honey, and lemon juice.
3. Simmer for 5-10 minutes until the mixture thickens.
4. Let cool before serving.

17. Lemon Poppy Seed Muffins

Ingredients:
- 1 cup almond flour
- 1/2 cup coconut flour
- 1/4 cup honey
- 3 eggs
- 1/4 cup coconut oil, melted
- 1 tbsp poppy seeds
- 1 tsp vanilla extract
- 1 tsp baking powder
- 1/4 tsp salt
- Zest of 1 lemon

Instructions:
1. Preheat the oven to 350°F (175°C).
2. In a bowl, mix almond flour, coconut flour, baking powder, and salt.
3. In another bowl, whisk eggs, honey, melted coconut oil, vanilla extract, and lemon zest.

4. Mix the wet and dry ingredients together thoroughly.

5. Fold in poppy seeds.

6. Divide batter into a muffin tin lined with paper liners.

7. Bake for 20-25 minutes until a toothpick inserted comes out clean.

18. Peanut Butter Banana Ice Cream

Ingredients:
- 4 ripe bananas, sliced and frozen
- 1/4 cup natural peanut butter
- 1 tsp vanilla extract

Instructions:
1. In a food processor, blend frozen banana slices until smooth.

2. Add peanut butter and vanilla extract, and blend until well combined.

3. Serve immediately or freeze for later.

19. Coconut Milk Panna Cotta

Ingredients:
- 1 can coconut milk
- 1/4 cup honey
- 1 tsp vanilla extract
- 1 packet gelatin
- Fresh berries for topping

Instructions:

1. In a small saucepan, heat coconut milk and honey over medium heat until warm.
2. Stir in vanilla extract.
3. In a separate bowl, dissolve gelatin in 2 tbsp of water.
4. Stir the gelatin mixture into the coconut milk until well combined.
5. Pour into serving dishes and refrigerate for at least 2 hours until set.
6. Serve topped with fresh berries.

20. Dark Chocolate Coconut Bites

Ingredients:
- 1 cup shredded coconut
- 1/4 cup coconut oil, melted
- 1/4 cup honey
- 1 cup dark chocolate chips

Instructions:

1. In a bowl, mix shredded coconut, melted coconut oil, and honey.
2. Form the mixture into small balls and place on a baking sheet lined with parchment paper.
3. Freeze for 30 minutes until firm.
4. Melt dark chocolate chips in a microwave-safe bowl, stirring every 30 seconds until smooth.

5. Dip the coconut balls in the melted chocolate and place back on the baking sheet.
6. Refrigerate until the chocolate is set.

21. Berry Chia Pudding

Ingredients:
- 1 cup almond milk
- 1/4 cup chia seeds
- 2 tbsp honey
- 1 tsp vanilla extract
- 1/2 cup mixed berries

Instructions:
1. In a bowl, mix almond milk, chia seeds, honey, and vanilla extract.
2. Cover and refrigerate overnight or for at least 4 hours.
3. Serve topped with mixed berries.

22. Baked Pears with Walnuts

Ingredients:
- 4 pears, halved and cored
- 1/4 cup chopped walnuts
- 2 tbsp honey
- 1 tsp ground cinnamon

Instructions:

1. Preheat the oven to 375°F (190°C).
2. Place pear halves in a baking dish.
3. In a small bowl, mix chopped walnuts, honey, and ground cinnamon.
4. Spoon the walnut mixture into the pear cavities.
5. Bake for 20-25 minutes until the pears are tender.

23. Carrot Cake Energy Bites

Ingredients:
- 1 cup rolled oats
- 1/2 cup grated carrots
- 1/4 cup almond butter
- 1/4 cup honey
- 1/2 cup shredded coconut
- 1 tsp ground cinnamon
- 1/2 tsp ground ginger
- 1/4 tsp ground nutmeg

Instructions:
1. In a large bowl, mix rolled oats, grated carrots, almond butter, honey, shredded coconut, ground cinnamon, ground ginger, and ground nutmeg.
2. Form the mixture into small balls.
3. Refrigerate for at least 30 minutes before serving.

24. Mango Coconut Chia Pudding

Ingredients:
- 1 cup coconut milk
- 1/4 cup chia seeds
- 2 tbsp honey
- 1/2 cup diced mango

Instructions:
1. In a bowl, mix coconut milk, chia seeds, and honey.
2. Cover and refrigerate overnight or for at least 4 hours.
3. Serve topped with diced mango.

25. Almond Butter Chocolate Bars

Ingredients:
- 1/2 cup almond butter
- 1/4 cup honey
- 1/4 cup coconut flour
- 1/4 cup dark chocolate chips

Instructions:
1. In a bowl, mix almond butter, honey, and coconut flour until well combined.
2. Press the mixture into a baking dish lined with parchment paper.
3. Melt dark chocolate chips in a microwave-safe bowl, stirring every 30 seconds until smooth.
4. Pour the melted chocolate over the almond butter mixture.

5. Refrigerate for at least 2 hours until set.
6. Cut into bars before serving.

26. Lemon Raspberry Chia Bars

Ingredients:
- 1 cup almond flour
- 1/2 cup coconut flour
- 1/4 cup honey
- 3 eggs
- 1/4 cup coconut oil, melted
- 1 cup raspberries
- 2 tbsp chia seeds
- 1 tsp vanilla extract
- 1 tsp baking powder
- 1/4 tsp salt
- Zest of 1 lemon

Instructions:
1. Preheat the oven to 350°F (175°C).
2. In a bowl, mix almond flour, coconut flour, baking powder, and salt.
3. In another bowl, whisk eggs, honey, melted coconut oil, vanilla extract, and lemon zest.
4. Combine wet and dry ingredients until well mixed.
5. Fold in raspberries and chia seeds.
6. Spread the batter into a baking dish lined with parchment paper.

7. Bake for 20-25 minutes until a toothpick inserted comes out clean.

27. Dark Chocolate Covered Strawberries

Ingredients:
- 1 cup dark chocolate chips
- 1 pint strawberries

Instructions:
1. Melt dark chocolate chips in a microwave-safe bowl, stirring every 30 seconds until smooth.
2. Dip each strawberry into the melted chocolate, then place on a baking sheet lined with parchment paper.
3. Refrigerate until the chocolate is set.

28. Almond Joy Bites

Ingredients:
- 1 cup shredded coconut
- 1/4 cup coconut oil, melted
- 1/4 cup honey
- 1/4 cup almonds, chopped
- 1/2 cup dark chocolate chips

Instructions:
1. In a bowl, mix shredded coconut, melted coconut oil, honey, and chopped almonds.

2. Form the mixture into small balls and place on a baking sheet lined with parchment paper.
3. Freeze for 30 minutes until firm.
4. Melt dark chocolate chips in a microwave-safe bowl, stirring every 30 seconds until smooth.
5. Dip the coconut balls in the melted chocolate and place back on the baking sheet.
6. Refrigerate until the chocolate is set.

29. Blueberry Almond Crumble

Ingredients:
- 2 cups blueberries
- 1 cup almond flour
- 1/4 cup chopped almonds
- 2 tbsp honey
- 2 tbsp coconut oil, melted
- 1 tsp vanilla extract
- Pinch of salt

Instructions:
1. Preheat the oven to 350°F (175°C).
2. Place blueberries in a baking dish.
3. In a bowl, mix almond flour, chopped almonds, honey, melted coconut oil, vanilla extract, and salt.
4. Sprinkle the crumble mixture over the blueberries.
5. Bake for 20-25 minutes until golden brown.

30. Chocolate Peanut Butter Chia Pudding

Ingredients:
- 1 cup almond milk
- 1/4 cup chia seeds
- 2 tbsp unsweetened cocoa powder
- 2 tbsp peanut butter
- 2 tbsp honey
- 1 tsp vanilla extract

Instructions:
1. In a bowl, mix almond milk, chia seeds, cocoa powder, peanut butter, honey, and vanilla extract.
2. Cover and refrigerate overnight or for at least 4 hours.
3. Serve chilled.

31. Cinnamon Apple Chips

Ingredients:
- 2 large apples, thinly sliced
- 1 tsp ground cinnamon

Instructions:
1. Preheat the oven to 225°F (110°C).
2. Arrange apple slices on a baking sheet lined with parchment paper.
3. Sprinkle it with ground cinnamon.

4. Bake for 1-2 hours until the apples are crisp, flipping halfway through.

32. Coconut Milk Mango Popsicles

Ingredients:
- 2 cups coconut milk
- 1 cup diced mango
- 2 tbsp honey
- 1 tsp vanilla extract

Instructions:
1. Blend coconut milk, diced mango, honey, and vanilla extract until smooth.
2. Pour the mixture into popsicle molds.
3. Freeze for at least 4 hours until set.

33. Dark Chocolate Avocado Brownies

Ingredients:
- 2 ripe avocados
- 1/2 cup unsweetened cocoa powder
- 1/2 cup honey
- 1/4 cup almond flour
- 2 eggs
- 1 tsp vanilla extract
- 1/2 tsp baking soda
- 1/4 tsp salt

Instructions:

1. Preheat the oven to 350°F (175°C).

2. In a bowl, blend avocados, cocoa powder, honey, almond flour, eggs, vanilla extract, baking soda, and salt until smooth.

3. Pour the batter into a greased baking pan.

4. Bake for 20-25 minutes until a toothpick inserted comes out clean.

34. Raspberry Coconut Chia Bars

Ingredients:
- 1 cup almond flour
- 1/2 cup coconut flour
- 1/4 cup honey
- 3 eggs
- 1/4 cup coconut oil, melted
- 1 cup raspberries
- 2 tbsp chia seeds
- 1 tsp vanilla extract
- 1 tsp baking powder
- 1/4 tsp salt

Instructions:

1. Preheat the oven to 350°F (175°C).

2. In a bowl, combine almond flour, coconut flour, baking powder, and salt.

3. In another bowl, whisk eggs, honey, melted coconut oil, and vanilla extract.
4. Combine the wet and dry ingredients until well mixed.
5. Fold in raspberries and chia seeds.
6. Spread the batter into a baking dish lined with parchment paper.
7. Bake for 20-25 minutes until a toothpick inserted comes out clean.

35. Lemon Poppy Seed Energy Bites

Ingredients:
- 1 cup rolled oats
- 1/4 cup almond butter
- 1/4 cup honey
- 1 tbsp poppy seeds
- 1 tsp vanilla extract
- Zest of 1 lemon

Instructions:
1. In a large bowl, mix rolled oats, almond butter, honey, poppy seeds, vanilla extract, and lemon zest.
2. Form the mixture into small balls.
3. Refrigerate for at least 30 minutes before serving.

36. Dark Chocolate Raspberry Bark

Ingredients:

- 1 cup dark chocolate chips
- 1/2 cup raspberries

Instructions:

1. Melt dark chocolate chips in a microwave-safe bowl, stirring every 30 seconds until smooth.
2. Spread the melted chocolate onto a baking sheet lined with parchment paper.
3. Sprinkle raspberries over the melted chocolate.
4. Refrigerate until set, then break into pieces.

37. Strawberry Chia Jam

Ingredients:
- 2 cups fresh strawberries
- 2 tbsp chia seeds
- 1-2 tbsp honey (optional)
- 1 tsp lemon juice

Instructions:

1. In a small saucepan, cook strawberries over medium heat until they begin to break down.
2. Mash the strawberries with a fork and stir in chia seeds, honey, and lemon juice.
3. Simmer for 5-10 minutes until the mixture thickens.
4. Let cool before serving.

38. Almond Butter Chocolate Chip Cookies

Ingredients:
- 1 cup almond butter
- 1/4 cup honey
- 1 egg
- 1/4 cup dark chocolate chips
- 1 tsp vanilla extract
- 1/2 tsp baking soda
- Pinch of salt

Instructions:
1. Preheat the oven to 350°F (175°C).
2. In a bowl, mix almond butter, honey, egg, dark chocolate chips, vanilla extract, baking soda, and salt.
3. Drop spoonfuls of dough onto a baking sheet lined with parchment paper.
4. Bake for 10-12 minutes until golden brown.

39. Banana Nut Muffins

Ingredients:
- 1 cup almond flour
- 1/2 cup coconut flour
- 1/4 cup honey
- 3 eggs
- 1/4 cup coconut oil, melted
- 1 ripe banana, mashed
- 1/4 cup chopped nuts (walnuts, pecans)

- 1 tsp vanilla extract
- 1 tsp baking powder
- 1/4 tsp salt

Instructions:
1. Preheat the oven to 350°F (175°C).
2. In a bowl, combine almond flour, coconut flour, baking powder, and salt.
3. In another bowl, whisk eggs, honey, melted coconut oil, mashed banana, and vanilla extract.
4. Combine the wet and dry ingredients until well mixed.
5. Fold in chopped nuts.
6. Divide batter into a muffin tin lined with paper liners.
7. Bake for 20-25 minutes until a toothpick inserted comes out clean.

40. Lemon Coconut Bars

Ingredients:
- 1 cup almond flour
- 1/2 cup shredded coconut
- 1/4 cup honey
- 3 eggs
- 1/4 cup coconut oil, melted
- 1 tsp vanilla extract
- 1 tsp baking powder
- 1/4 tsp salt
- Zest of 1 lemon

Instructions:

1. Preheat the oven to 350°F (175°C).

2. In a bowl, mix almond flour, shredded coconut, baking powder, and salt.

3. In another bowl, whisk eggs, honey, melted coconut oil, vanilla extract, and lemon zest.

4. Combine the wet and dry ingredients until well mixed.

5. Spread the batter into a baking dish lined with parchment paper.

6. Bake for 20-25 minutes until a toothpick inserted comes out clean.

41. Dark Chocolate Peanut Butter Cups

Ingredients:
- 1 cup dark chocolate chips
- 1/2 cup natural peanut butter
- 2 tbsp coconut oil, melted
- 1 tsp vanilla extract
- Pinch of salt

Instructions:

1. Melt dark chocolate chips in a microwave-safe bowl, stirring every 30 seconds until smooth.

2. In another bowl, mix peanut butter, melted coconut oil, vanilla extract, and salt.

3. Line a muffin tin with paper liners.

4. Spoon a small amount of melted chocolate into each liner.

5. Freeze for 10 minutes until chocolate is set.

6. Spoon peanut butter mixture over the chocolate layer.

7. Top with another layer of melted chocolate.

8. Freeze until fully set.

42. Blueberry Almond Bars

Ingredients:
- 1 cup almond flour
- 1/2 cup coconut flour
- 1/4 cup honey
- 3 eggs
- 1/4 cup coconut oil, melted
- 1 cup blueberries
- 1 tsp vanilla extract
- 1 tsp baking powder
- 1/4 tsp salt

Instructions:
1. Preheat the oven to 350°F (175°C).

2. In a bowl, mix almond flour, coconut flour, baking powder, and salt.

3. In another bowl, whisk eggs, honey, melted coconut oil, and vanilla extract.

4. Combine the wet and dry ingredients until well mixed.

5. Fold in blueberries.

6. Spread the batter into a baking dish lined with parchment paper.

7. Bake for 20-25 minutes until a toothpick inserted comes out clean.

43. Chocolate Coconut Mousse

Ingredients:
- 1 can coconut milk
- 1/4 cup unsweetened cocoa powder
- 1/4 cup honey
- 1 tsp vanilla extract

Instructions:
1. Chill the can of coconut milk in the refrigerator overnight.

2. Scoop the solidified coconut cream into a bowl, leaving the liquid behind.

3. Add cocoa powder, honey, and vanilla extract to the coconut cream.

4. Whip with a mixer until light and fluffy.

5. Serve immediately or refrigerate for later.

44. Lemon Blueberry Chia Pudding

Ingredients:
- 1 cup almond milk
- 1/4 cup chia seeds

- 2 tbsp honey
- 1 tsp vanilla extract
- 1/2 cup blueberries
- Zest of 1 lemon

Instructions:

1. In a bowl, mix almond milk, chia seeds, honey, vanilla extract, blueberries, and lemon zest.
2. Cover and refrigerate overnight or for at least 4 hours.
3. Serve chilled.

45. Dark Chocolate Almond Clusters

Ingredients:
- 1 cup dark chocolate chips
- 1/2 cup almonds

Instructions:

1. Melt dark chocolate chips in a microwave-safe bowl, stirring every 30 seconds until smooth.
2. Stir in almonds until well coated.
3. Use a spoon to place dollops of dough onto a baking sheet lined with parchment paper.
4. Refrigerate until set.

46. Raspberry Coconut Energy Bites

Ingredients:

- 1 cup rolled oats
- 1/4 cup almond butter
- 1/4 cup honey
- 1/2 cup shredded coconut
- 1/2 cup raspberries
- 1 tsp vanilla extract

Instructions:

1. In a large bowl, mix rolled oats, almond butter, honey, shredded coconut, raspberries, and vanilla extract until well combined.
2. Form the mixture into small balls.
3. Refrigerate for at least 30 minutes before serving.

47. Chocolate Covered Banana Slices

Ingredients:
- 2 ripe bananas, sliced
- 1/2 cup dark chocolate chips
- 1 tsp coconut oil
- Chopped nuts or shredded coconut for topping (optional)

Instructions:

1. Line a baking sheet with parchment paper.
2. Place banana slices on the baking sheet.
3. In a microwave-safe bowl, melt dark chocolate chips with coconut oil, stirring every 30 seconds until smooth.

4. Dip each banana slice halfway into the melted chocolate and place back on the baking sheet.
5. Sprinkle with chopped nuts or shredded coconut if desired.
6. Freeze for 1-2 hours until chocolate is set.

48. Almond Joy Chia Pudding

Ingredients:
- 1 cup almond milk
- 1/4 cup chia seeds
- 2 tbsp honey
- 2 tbsp unsweetened shredded coconut
- 2 tbsp sliced almonds
- 1 tbsp cocoa powder
- 1/2 tsp vanilla extract

Instructions:
1. In a bowl, mix almond milk, chia seeds, honey, shredded coconut, sliced almonds, cocoa powder, and vanilla extract.
2. Cover and refrigerate overnight or for at least 4 hours.
3. Serve chilled.

49. Coconut Flour Pancakes

Ingredients:
- 1/4 cup coconut flour

- 2 tbsp almond flour
- 2 eggs
- 1/4 cup almond milk
- 2 tbsp honey
- 1/2 tsp baking powder
- 1/4 tsp vanilla extract
- Pinch of salt
- Coconut oil for cooking

Instructions:

1. In a bowl, whisk together coconut flour, almond flour, baking powder, and salt.
2. In another bowl, beat eggs, almond milk, honey, and vanilla extract until well combined.
3. Gradually add the wet ingredients to the dry ingredients and mix until smooth.
4. Heat coconut oil in a skillet over medium heat.
5. Pour approximately 1/4 cup of batter onto the skillet for each pancake.
6. Cook until bubbles start to appear on the surface, then carefully flip and cook until the other side turns a golden brown hue.
7. Serve warm with your favorite toppings.

50. Strawberry Banana Smoothie Bowl

Ingredients:

- 1 frozen banana

- 1/2 cup frozen strawberries
- 1/4 cup almond milk
- 1/4 cup Greek yogurt
- 1 tbsp honey
- Toppings: sliced strawberries, sliced bananas, shredded coconut, granola, chia seeds

Instructions:

1. In a blender, combine frozen banana, frozen strawberries, almond milk, Greek yogurt, and honey until smooth.
2. Pour the smoothie into a bowl.
3. Top with sliced strawberries, sliced bananas, shredded coconut, granola, and chia seeds.
4. Serve immediately.

50 nutrient-dense low glycemic snack recipes:

1. Greek Yogurt with Berries
- **Ingredients:**
- 1/2 cup Greek yogurt
- Mixed berries (such as strawberries, blueberries, raspberries)
- **Instructions:**
1. Place Greek yogurt in a bowl.

2. Top with mixed berries.

3. Enjoy!

2. Almond Butter Apple Slices

- Ingredients:

- 1 apple, sliced

- 2 tbsp almond butter

- Instructions:

  1. Spread almond butter on apple slices.

  2. Enjoy as a crunchy and creamy snack.

3. Carrot Sticks with Hummus

- Ingredients:

- Carrot sticks

- Hummus

- Instructions:

  1. Dip carrot sticks into hummus.

  2. Enjoy the crunchy texture with creamy hummus.

4. Celery with Peanut Butter

- Ingredients:

- Celery sticks

- Peanut butter

- Instructions:

  1. Spread peanut butter on celery sticks.

  2. Enjoy as a satisfying and crunchy snack.

5. Cottage Cheese with Pineapple

- Ingredients:

- 1/2 cup cottage cheese
- Fresh pineapple chunks

- Instructions:

1. Serve cottage cheese topped with fresh pineapple chunks.
2. Enjoy the creamy and sweet combination.

6. Hard-Boiled Eggs

- Ingredients:

- Eggs

- Instructions:

   1. Hard-boil eggs until cooked.
   2. Peel and enjoy as a protein-rich snack.

7. Avocado Toast

- Ingredients:

- Whole grain bread
- Avocado
- Salt and pepper (optional)

- Instructions:

   1. Toast whole grain bread.
   2. Spread mashed avocado on top.
   3. Season with salt and pepper if desired.
   4. Enjoy as a simple and nutritious snack.

8. Trail Mix

- Ingredients:

- Mixed nuts (almonds, walnuts, cashews)
- Dried fruits (raisins, cranberries)
- Pumpkin seeds
- **Instructions:**
  1. Mix all ingredients together in a bowl.
  2. Portion into small servings for an easy grab-and-go snack.

9. Kale Chips
- **Ingredients:**
- Fresh kale leaves
- Olive oil
- Sea Salt
- **Instructions:**
  1. Preheat the oven to 350°F (175°C).
  2. Remove stems from kale leaves and tear into bite-sized pieces.
  3. Drizzle with olive oil and sprinkle with salt.
  4. Bake for 10-15 minutes until crispy.
  5. Enjoy as a crunchy and nutritious snack.

10. Edamame
- **Ingredients:**
- Edamame (fresh or frozen)
- Sea salt (optional)
- **Instructions:**
  1. Boil or steam edamame until tender.
  2. Sprinkle with sea salt if desired.

3. Enjoy by popping the beans out of the pods.

11. Cucumber Slices with Tzatziki
- Ingredients:
- Cucumber slices
- Tzatziki sauce

- Instructions:
   1. Dip cucumber slices into tzatziki sauce.
   2. Enjoy the cool and refreshing taste.

12. Cherry Tomatoes with Mozzarella
- Ingredients:
- Cherry tomatoes
- Fresh mozzarella balls
- Basil leaves (optional)

- Instructions:
   1. Thread cherry tomatoes, mozzarella balls, and basil leaves onto toothpicks.
   2. Enjoy as a flavorful and bite-sized snack.

13. Whole Grain Crackers with Cheese
- Ingredients:
- Whole grain crackers
- Cheese slices or cubes

- Instructions:
   1. Serve whole grain crackers with cheese.
   2. Enjoy as a satisfying and crunchy snack.

14. Almonds

- **Ingredients:**
- Almonds
- **Instructions:**

1. Enjoy a handful of almonds as a protein-packed snack.

15. Rice Cakes with Avocado and Tomato

- **Ingredients:**
- Rice cakes
- Avocado
- Tomato slices
- **Instructions:**

1. Spread mashed avocado on rice cakes.
2. Top with tomato slices.
3. Enjoy as a light and flavorful snack.

16. Bell Pepper Strips with Guacamole

- **Ingredients:**
- Bell pepper strips (assorted colors)
- Guacamole
- **Instructions:**

1. Dip bell pepper strips into guacamole.
2. Enjoy as a crunchy and creamy snack.

17. Cottage Cheese with Sliced Peaches

- **Ingredients:**
- 1/2 cup cottage cheese

- Fresh peach slices
- **Instructions:**
   1. Serve cottage cheese topped with fresh peach slices.
   2. Enjoy the creamy and sweet combination.

18. Almond Flour Crackers with Goat Cheese
- **Ingredients:**
- Almond flour crackers
- Goat cheese
- **Instructions:**
   1. Spread goat cheese onto almond flour crackers.
   2. Enjoy as a flavorful and satisfying snack.

19. Veggie Sticks with Guacamole
- **Ingredients:**
- Assorted veggie sticks (carrots, celery, bell peppers)
- Guacamole
- **Instructions:**
   1. Dip veggie sticks into guacamole.
   2. Enjoy as a crunchy and nutritious snack.

20. Popcorn
- **Ingredients:**
- Popcorn kernels
- Olive oil
- Sea salt (optional)
- **Instructions:**

1. Pop popcorn kernels using an air popper or stovetop method.

2. Drizzle with olive oil and sprinkle with sea salt if desired.

3. Enjoy as a light and satisfying snack.

21. Turkey Roll-Ups

- Ingredients:

- Sliced turkey breast

- Spinach leaves

- Mustard (optional)

- Instructions:

1. Place spinach leaves on top of turkey slices.

2. Roll up and secure with toothpicks.

3. Add mustard for extra flavor if desired.

4. Enjoy as a protein-rich snack.

22. Egg Muffins

- Ingredients:

- Eggs

- Spinach

- Cherry tomatoes

- Feta cheese (optional)

- Instructions:

1. Whisk eggs in a bowl and season with salt and pepper.

2. Stir in chopped spinach, halved cherry tomatoes, and crumbled feta cheese if using.

3. Pour mixture into muffin tins and bake at 350°F (175°C) for 20-25 minutes.

4. Let cool before enjoying as a protein-packed snack.

23. Chia Seed Pudding

- Ingredients:

- Chia seeds
- Almond milk
- Vanilla extract
- Honey (optional)

- Instructions:

1. Mix chia seeds, almond milk, vanilla extract, and honey in a bowl.

2. Refrigerate for at least 2 hours or overnight until thickened.

3. Enjoy chilled as a creamy and nutritious snack.

24. Cottage Cheese with Berries

- Ingredients:

- 1/2 cup cottage cheese
- Mixed berries (such as strawberries, blueberries, raspberries)

- Instructions:

1. Serve cottage cheese topped with mixed berries.

2. Enjoy the creamy and fruity combination.

25. Almond Flour Muffins

- Ingredients:

- Almond flour
- Eggs
- Honey
- Baking powder
- Vanilla extract
- **Instructions:**
   1. Mix almond flour, eggs, honey, baking powder, and vanilla extract in a bowl.
   2. Pour batter into muffin tins and bake at 350°F (175°C) for 20-25 minutes.
   3. Let cool before enjoying as a moist and satisfying snack.

26. Spinach and Artichoke Dip with Veggie Chips
- **Ingredients:**
- Spinach and artichoke dip
- Veggie chips
- **Instructions:**
   1. Dip veggie chips into spinach and artichoke dip.
   2. Enjoy as a flavorful and crunchy snack.

27. Zucchini Chips
- **Ingredients:**
- Zucchini, thinly sliced
- Olive oil
- Parmesan cheese (optional)
- **Instructions:**
   1. Preheat the oven to 225°F (110°C).

2. Toss zucchini slices with olive oil and sprinkle with Parmesan cheese if desired.

3. Bake for 1-2 hours until crispy.

4. Enjoy as a crunchy and savory snack.

28. Guacamole Deviled Eggs

- **Ingredients:**
- Hard-boiled eggs
- Avocado
- Lime juice
- Salt and pepper
- **Instructions:**

1. Cut hard-boiled eggs in half and remove yolks.

2. Mash yolks with avocado, lime juice, salt, and pepper.

3. Spoon mixture into egg whites.

4. Enjoy as a creamy and protein-rich snack.

29. Almond Flour Banana Bread

- **Ingredients:**
- Almond flour
- Ripe bananas
- Eggs
- Honey
- Baking soda
- Vanilla extract
- **Instructions:**

1. Mix almond flour, mashed bananas, eggs, honey, baking soda, and vanilla extract in a bowl.

2. Pour batter into a loaf pan and bake at 350°F (175°C) for 40-45 minutes.

3. Let cool before slicing and enjoying as a moist and flavorful snack.

30. Greek Yogurt Parfait

- Ingredients:
  - Greek yogurt
  - Granola
  - Fresh berries (such as strawberries, blueberries)

- Instructions:

1. Layer Greek yogurt, granola, and fresh berries in a glass.

2. Repeat layers if desired.

3. Enjoy as a creamy and crunchy snack.

31. Stuffed Bell Peppers with Quinoa and Black Beans

- Ingredients:
  - Bell peppers
  - Quinoa, cooked
  - Black beans, cooked
  - Salsa

- Instructions:

1. Cut tops off bell peppers and remove seeds.

2. Stuff peppers with cooked quinoa, black beans, and salsa.

3. Bake at 375°F (190°C) for 25-30 minutes.

4. Enjoy as a satisfying and flavorful snack.

32. Coconut Flour Banana Muffins

- Ingredients:
   - Coconut flour
   - Ripe bananas
   - Eggs
   - Honey
   - Baking powder
   - Vanilla extract

- Instructions:

1. Mix coconut flour, mashed bananas, eggs, honey, baking powder, and vanilla extract in a bowl.

2. Pour batter into muffin tins and bake at 350°F (175°C) for 20-25 minutes.

3. Let cool before enjoying as a moist and delicious snack.

33. Caprese Skewers

- Ingredients:
   - Cherry tomatoes
   - Fresh mozzarella balls
   - Basil leaves
   - Balsamic glaze (optional)

- Instructions:

1. Thread cherry tomatoes, fresh mozzarella balls, and basil leaves onto toothpicks.

2. Drizzle with balsamic glaze if desired.

3. Enjoy as a flavorful and bite-sized snack.

34. Sweet Potato Chips

- Ingredients:

- Sweet potatoes, thinly sliced
- Olive oil
- Sea salt

- Instructions:

1. Preheat the oven to 225°F (110°C).

2. Toss sweet potato slices with olive oil and sprinkle with sea salt.

3. Bake for 1-2 hours until crispy.

4. Enjoy as a crunchy and nutritious snack.

35. Greek Yogurt Bark

- Ingredients:

- Greek yogurt
- Mixed berries (such as strawberries, blueberries, raspberries)
- Honey

- Instructions:

1. Line a baking sheet with parchment paper.

2. Spread Greek yogurt onto parchment paper.

3. Top with mixed berries and drizzle with honey.

4. Freeze until firm, then break into pieces.

5. Enjoy as a creamy and fruity snack.

36. Turkey Jerky
- **Ingredients:**
  - Turkey breast, thinly sliced
  - Soy sauce
  - Worcestershire sauce
  - Garlic powder
  - Onion powder
- **Instructions:**

1. Marinate turkey slices in soy sauce, Worcestershire sauce, garlic powder, and onion powder for 1 hour.

2. Dehydrate in a food dehydrator or oven at a low temperature until dry and chewy.

3. Enjoy as a protein-rich and portable snack.

37. Baked Apple Chips
- **Ingredients:**
  - Apples, thinly sliced
  - Cinnamon
- **Instructions:**

1. Preheat the oven to 225°F (110°C).

2. Arrange apple slices on a baking sheet lined with parchment paper.

3. Sprinkle with cinnamon.

4. Bake for 1-2 hours until crispy.

5. Enjoy as a sweet and crunchy snack.

38. Spinach and Feta Stuffed Mushrooms

- Ingredients:
  - Mushrooms
  - Spinach, chopped
  - Feta cheese, crumbled
  - Garlic, minced

- Instructions:
  1. Remove stems from mushrooms and place caps on a baking sheet.
  2. Mix chopped spinach, crumbled feta cheese, and minced garlic in a bowl.
  3. Stuffed mushroom caps with spinach and feta mixture.
  4. Bake at 375°F (190°C) for 15-20 minutes.
  5. Enjoy as a flavorful and savory snack.

39. Quinoa Salad Cups

- Ingredients:
  - Cooked quinoa
  - Cucumber, diced
  - Cherry tomatoes, halved
  - Red onion, diced
  - Feta cheese, crumbled
  - Lemon juice
  - Olive oil
  - Fresh parsley, chopped

- Instructions:

1. Mix cooked quinoa, diced cucumber, halved cherry tomatoes, diced red onion, crumbled feta cheese, lemon juice, olive oil, and chopped fresh parsley in a bowl.

2. Spoon mixture into lettuce cups or endive leaves.

3. Enjoy as a refreshing and nutrient-dense snack.

40. Stuffed Dates

- Ingredients:

- Medjool dates, pitted
- Almond butter
- Walnuts

- Instructions:

1. Fill each date with almond butter and top with a walnut.

2. Enjoy as a sweet and satisfying snack.

41. Cucumber Slices with Smoked Salmon

- Ingredients:

- Cucumber slices
- Smoked salmon

- Instructions:

1. Place smoked salmon on top of cucumber slices.

2. Enjoy as a refreshing and protein-rich snack.

42. Cauliflower Hummus

- Ingredients:

- Cauliflower, chopped
- Olive oil

- Tahini
- Lemon juice
- Garlic
- Cumin
- **Instructions:**
   1. Roast chopped cauliflower with olive oil until tender.
   2. Blend roasted cauliflower with tahini, lemon juice, garlic, and cumin until smooth.
   3. Serve with veggie sticks or whole grain crackers.
   4. Enjoy as a creamy and flavorful snack.

43. Turkey and Cheese Roll-Ups
- **Ingredients:**
   - Sliced turkey breast
   - Cheese slices
- **Instructions:**
   1. Place cheese slices on top of turkey slices.
   2. Roll up and enjoy as a protein-rich snack.

44. Roasted Chickpeas
- **Ingredients:**
   - Chickpeas (canned or cooked)
   - Olive oil
   - Seasonings (such as paprika, garlic powder, cumin)
- **Instructions:**
   1. Toss chickpeas with olive oil and seasonings.
   2. Roast in the oven at 400°F (200°C) for 20-30 minutes until crispy.

3. Enjoy as a crunchy and fiber-rich snack.

45. Seaweed Snacks
- **Ingredients:**
  - Roasted seaweed sheets
- **Instructions:**
  1. Enjoy roasted seaweed sheets as a light and flavorful snack.

46. Broccoli and Cheese Bites
- **Ingredients:**
  - Broccoli florets
  - Cheddar cheese, shredded
  - Eggs
  - Almond flour
- **Instructions:**
  1. Steam broccoli florets until tender.
  2. Mash broccoli and mix with shredded cheddar cheese, eggs, and almond flour.
  3. Form into bite-sized balls and bake at 375°F (190°C) for 15-20 minutes.
  4. Enjoy as a cheesy and nutritious snack.

47. Beet Chips
- **Ingredients:**
  - Beets, thinly sliced
  - Olive oil
  - Sea salt

- **Instructions:**
  1. Preheat the oven to 350°F (175°C).
  2. Toss beet slices with olive oil and sprinkle with sea salt.
  3. Bake for 20-25 minutes until crispy.
  4. Enjoy as a colorful and crunchy snack.

48. Chocolate Avocado Pudding
- **Ingredients:**
  - Avocado
  - Cocoa powder
  - Honey
  - Almond milk
- **Instructions:**
  1. Blend avocado, cocoa powder, honey, and almond milk until smooth.
  2. Chill in the refrigerator for at least 30 minutes.
  3. Enjoy as a creamy and decadent snack.

49. Eggplant Chips
- **Ingredients:**
  - Eggplant, thinly sliced
  - Olive oil
  - Italian seasoning
- **Instructions:**
  1. Preheat the oven to 375°F (190°C).
  2. Toss eggplant slices with olive oil and Italian seasoning.

3. Bake for 20-25 minutes until crispy.

4. Enjoy as a savory and crispy snack.

50. Cucumber Cups with Tuna Salad
- **Ingredients:**
  - Cucumber, sliced into thick rounds
  - Canned tuna, drained
  - Greek yogurt
  - Dijon mustard
  - Dill
- **Instructions:**
  1. Scoop out a small portion of the center of each cucumber round to create a cup.
  2. Mix canned tuna, Greek yogurt, Dijon mustard, and dill in a bowl.
  3. Fill cucumber cups with tuna salad.
  4. Enjoy as a refreshing and protein-rich snack.

With these 100 nutrient-dense, low glycemic desserts and snacks, you'll never have to compromise on taste or nutrition again. Whether you're craving something sweet, savory, or somewhere in between, there's a recipe here to satisfy every craving while supporting your health and wellness goals. Enjoy!

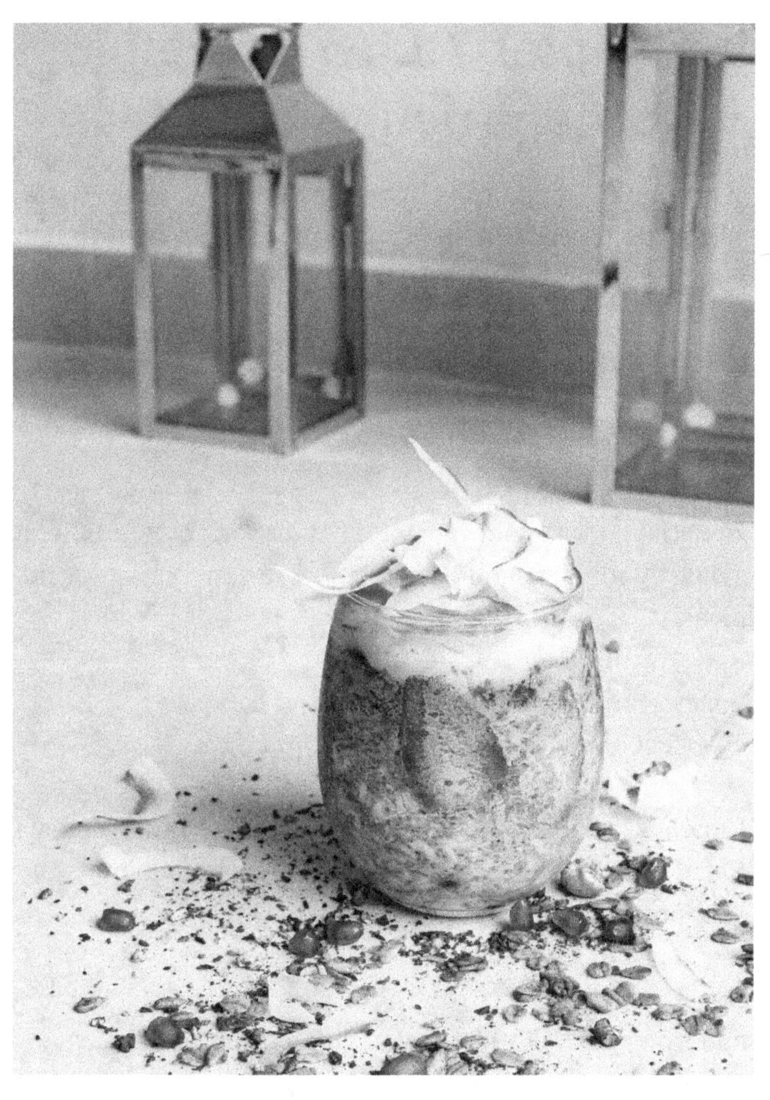

Chapter 7:Low Glycemic Nutrient-dense Meal Plan

Welcome to your Low Glycemic Nutrient-Dense 30-Day Meal Plan! This comprehensive plan is designed to help you maintain stable blood sugar levels, promote overall health, and satisfy your taste buds with delicious meals, snacks, and desserts. Let's dive in!

Day 1

Breakfast: Start your day with a nutritious bowl of Greek Yogurt with Berries for a creamy and satisfying morning meal.

Snack: Enjoy the crunch of Almond Butter Apple Slices, a perfect blend of sweetness and protein.

Lunch: Fuel your midday with a refreshing Spinach Salad with Grilled Chicken, packed with vitamins and lean protein.

Snack: Dive into Carrot Sticks with Hummus, a crunchy and savory snack to keep you going until dinner.

Dinner: Indulge in the delightful flavors of Baked Salmon with Roasted Vegetables, providing omega-3 fatty acids and a rainbow of nutrients.

Dessert: Treat yourself to a guilt-free Chia Seed Pudding, offering a creamy texture and a hint of sweetness to end your day on a high note.

Day 2

Breakfast: Wake up to the fluffy goodness of Almond Flour Pancakes, paired with your favorite toppings for a delightful start to the day.

Snack: Dive into Cottage Cheese with Pineapple, a creamy and tropical snack that satisfies your cravings.

Lunch: Enjoy the refreshing flavors of Quinoa Salad Cups, bursting with protein and fiber to keep you satisfied until your next meal.

Snack: Grab a handful of Trail Mix, offering a mix of nuts, seeds, and dried fruits for a satisfying crunch.

Dinner: Savor the hearty goodness of Stuffed Bell Peppers with Quinoa and Black Beans, a colorful and nutritious meal that's as satisfying as it is delicious.

Dessert: Treat yourself to Coconut Flour Banana Muffins, a moist and flavorful dessert that's perfect for satisfying your sweet tooth.

Day 3

Breakfast: Kickstart your morning with the simplicity of Avocado Toast, offering a creamy and flavorful base for your favorite toppings.

Snack: Enjoy the convenience of Hard-Boiled Eggs, providing a protein-packed snack to keep you energized throughout the day.

Lunch: Delight in the convenience of Turkey Roll-Ups with Spinach, offering a satisfying blend of protein and greens in every bite.

Snack: Indulge in the creamy goodness of Greek Yogurt Parfait, layered with granola and fresh berries for a sweet and satisfying snack.

Dinner: Dive into the savory flavors of Cauliflower Hummus with Veggie Sticks, offering a nutritious and flavorful alternative to traditional dips.

Dessert: Treat yourself to the creamy indulgence of Greek Yogurt Bark, offering a satisfyingly sweet treat to end your day on a high note.

Day 4

Breakfast: Start your day on a high note with Whole Grain Crackers with Cheese, offering a satisfying blend of fiber and protein to keep you feeling full and satisfied.

Snack: Enjoy the crunchy goodness of Kale Chips, offering a nutritious and flavorful alternative to traditional potato chips.

Lunch: Dig into the refreshing flavors of Zucchini Noodles with Pesto, offering a light and flavorful alternative to traditional pasta dishes.

Snack: Satisfy your sweet tooth with Cottage Cheese with Berries, offering a creamy and refreshing treat that's perfect for any time of day.

Dinner: Indulge in the savory goodness of Turkey and Cheese Roll-Ups, offering a satisfying blend of protein and cheese in every bite.

Dessert: Treat yourself to the rich and creamy goodness of Chocolate Avocado Pudding, offering a satisfyingly sweet treat that's perfect for satisfying your sweet tooth.

Day 5

Breakfast: Start your day with the simplicity of Rice Cakes with Avocado and Tomato, offering a satisfying blend of creamy avocado and juicy tomato on a crunchy rice cake.

Snack: Enjoy the satisfying crunch of Roasted Chickpeas, offering a nutritious and flavorful alternative to traditional snack foods.

Lunch: Dig into the refreshing flavors of Greek Salad with Grilled Shrimp, offering a light and flavorful alternative to traditional lunch options.

Snack: Satisfy your cravings with the savory goodness of Beet Chips, offering a nutritious and flavorful alternative to traditional potato chips.

Dinner: Indulge in the hearty goodness of Cucumber Cups with Tuna Salad, offering a satisfying blend of protein and veggies in every bite.

Dessert: Treat yourself to the sweet and satisfying goodness of Stuffed Dates, offering a satisfyingly sweet treat that's perfect for any time of day.

Day 6

Breakfast: Indulge in the refreshing flavors of a Strawberry Banana Smoothie Bowl, packed with fruity goodness and topped with your favorite toppings for added crunch.

Snack: Keep your energy levels up with a handful of Almonds, offering a satisfying blend of protein, healthy fats, and fiber.

Lunch: Dive into the savory goodness of Eggplant Parmesan with Mixed Greens, offering a satisfying blend of cheesy goodness and leafy greens.

Snack: Grab a pack of Turkey Jerky for a convenient and protein-packed snack to keep you fueled throughout the day.

Dinner: Savor the delightful flavors of Cucumber Slices with Smoked Salmon, offering a refreshing and protein-rich meal that's perfect for any time of day.

Dessert: End your day on a sweet note with a creamy and indulgent serving of Chia Seed Pudding, offering a satisfyingly sweet treat to satisfy your cravings.

Day 7

Breakfast: Wake up to the delightful flavors of Chocolate Covered Banana Slices, offering a sweet and satisfying start to your day.

Snack: Enjoy the light and airy crunch of Popcorn, offering a satisfyingly salty and crunchy snack that's perfect for any time of day.

Lunch: Delight in the savory goodness of Spinach and Feta Stuffed Mushrooms, offering a flavorful and nutritious meal that's perfect for lunchtime.

Snack: Keep your energy levels up with a serving of Turkey Jerky, offering a convenient and protein-packed snack to keep you fueled throughout the day.

Dinner: Indulge in the hearty goodness of Broccoli and Cheese Bites, offering a satisfying blend of cheesy goodness and nutritious veggies.

Dessert: Treat yourself to a savory and satisfying serving of Cucumber Slices with Smoked Salmon, offering a refreshing and protein-rich dessert option.

Day 8

Breakfast: Start your day on a sweet note with a stack of fluffy and delicious Coconut Flour Pancakes, offering a satisfying blend of sweetness and texture.

Snack: Enjoy the creamy and tropical flavors of Cottage Cheese with Sliced Peaches, offering a refreshing and protein-packed snack that's perfect for any time of day.

Lunch: Dive into the refreshing goodness of Beet Chips, offering a satisfyingly crunchy and nutritious snack that's perfect for on-the-go.

Snack: Satisfy your cravings with the creamy and indulgent goodness of Guacamole Deviled Eggs, offering a savory and satisfying treat that's perfect for any time of day.

Dinner: Indulge in the savory goodness of Spinach and Feta Stuffed Mushrooms, offering a flavorful and nutritious meal that's perfect for any time of day.

Dessert: Treat yourself to a sweet and satisfying serving of Chocolate Covered Banana Slices, offering a deliciously decadent treat to satisfy your sweet tooth.

Day 9

Breakfast: Wake up to the delightful flavors of a savory and satisfying serving of Egg Muffins, offering a convenient and protein-packed breakfast option that's perfect for busy mornings.

Snack: Keep your energy levels up with a satisfying blend of Trail Mix, offering a deliciously crunchy and satisfying snack that's perfect for any time of day.

Lunch: Delight in the refreshing flavors of Sweet Potato Chips, offering a satisfyingly crunchy and nutritious snack that's perfect for on-the-go.

Snack: Keep your energy levels up with a satisfying blend of Greek Yogurt with Berries, offering a deliciously creamy and satisfying snack that's perfect for any time of day.

Dinner: Indulge in the hearty goodness of Roasted Chickpeas, offering a savory and satisfying snack that's perfect for any time of day.

Dessert: Treat yourself to a sweet and satisfying serving of Chocolate Avocado Pudding, offering a deliciously creamy and indulgent dessert option that's perfect for any time of day.

Day 10

Breakfast: Start your day on a sweet note with the delightful flavors of Greek Yogurt Parfait, offering a deliciously creamy and satisfying breakfast option that's perfect for any time of day.

Snack: Keep your energy levels up with a satisfying blend of Almonds, offering a deliciously crunchy and satisfying snack that's perfect for any time of day.

Lunch: Delight in the refreshing flavors of Bell Pepper Strips with Guacamole, offering a satisfyingly crunchy and nutritious snack that's perfect for any time of day.

Snack: Keep your energy levels up with a satisfying blend of Seaweed Snacks, offering a deliciously savory and satisfying snack that's perfect for any time of day.

Dinner: Indulge in the hearty goodness of Cucumber Cups with Tuna Salad, offering a refreshing and protein-packed meal that's perfect for any time of day.

Dessert: Treat yourself to a sweet and satisfying serving of Almond Butter Apple Slices, offering a deliciously crunchy and satisfying dessert option that's perfect for any time of day.

Day 11

Breakfast: Kickstart your morning with the refreshing flavors of a Strawberry Banana Smoothie Bowl, topped with granola and fresh fruit for added texture and sweetness.

Snack: Keep your energy levels up with a handful of Almonds, offering a satisfying blend of protein and healthy fats to keep you fueled throughout the day.

Lunch: Delight in the savory goodness of Eggplant Parmesan with Mixed Greens, offering a satisfying blend of cheesy goodness and nutritious veggies.

Snack: Satisfy your cravings with the savory goodness of Turkey Jerky, offering a convenient and protein-packed snack to keep you going until dinner.

Dinner: Indulge in the hearty flavors of Cucumber Slices with Smoked Salmon, offering a refreshing and protein-rich meal that's perfect for any time of day.

Dessert: Treat yourself to a creamy and indulgent serving of Chia Seed Pudding, offering a satisfyingly sweet treat to end your day on a high note.

Day 12

Breakfast: Start your day with a stack of fluffy and flavorful Coconut Flour Pancakes, topped with fresh berries and a drizzle of honey for a sweet and satisfying breakfast.

Snack: Enjoy the creamy goodness of Cottage Cheese with Sliced Peaches, offering a refreshing and protein-packed snack to keep you fueled throughout the day.

Lunch: Dive into the refreshing flavors of Beet Chips, offering a satisfyingly crunchy and nutritious snack that's perfect for on-the-go.

Snack: Satisfy your sweet tooth with the indulgent flavors of Guacamole Deviled Eggs, offering a savory and satisfying treat that's perfect for any time of day.

Dinner: Indulge in the savory goodness of Spinach and Feta Stuffed Mushrooms, offering a flavorful and nutritious meal that's perfect for any time of day.

Dessert: Treat yourself to the sweet and satisfying goodness of Chocolate Covered Banana Slices, offering a deliciously decadent treat to satisfy your cravings.

Day 13

Breakfast: Wake up to the delightful flavors of a savory and satisfying serving of Egg Muffins, offering a convenient and protein-packed breakfast option that's perfect for busy mornings.

Snack: Keep your energy levels up with a satisfying blend of Trail Mix, offering a deliciously crunchy and satisfying snack that's perfect for any time of day.

Lunch: Delight in the refreshing flavors of Sweet Potato Chips, offering a satisfyingly crunchy and nutritious snack that's perfect for on-the-go.

Snack: Keep your energy levels up with a satisfying blend of Greek Yogurt with Berries, offering a deliciously creamy and satisfying snack that's perfect for any time of day.

Dinner: Indulge in the hearty goodness of Roasted Chickpeas, offering a savory and satisfying snack that's perfect for any time of day.

Dessert: Treat yourself to a sweet and satisfying serving of Chocolate Avocado Pudding, offering a deliciously creamy and indulgent dessert option that's perfect for any time of day.

Day 14

Breakfast: Start your day on a sweet note with the delightful flavors of Greek Yogurt Parfait, offering a deliciously creamy and satisfying breakfast option that's perfect for any time of day.

Snack: Keep your energy levels up with a satisfying blend of Almonds, offering a deliciously crunchy and satisfying snack that's perfect for any time of day.

Lunch: Delight in the refreshing flavors of Bell Pepper Strips with Guacamole, offering a satisfyingly crunchy and nutritious snack that's perfect for any time of day.

Snack: Keep your energy levels up with a satisfying blend of Seaweed Snacks, offering a deliciously savory and satisfying snack that's perfect for any time of day.

Dinner: Indulge in the hearty goodness of Cucumber Cups with Tuna Salad, offering a refreshing and protein-packed meal that's perfect for any time of day.

Dessert: Treat yourself to a sweet and satisfying serving of Almond Butter Apple Slices, offering a deliciously crunchy and satisfying dessert option that's perfect for any time of day.

Day 15

Breakfast: Enjoy a hearty and filling serving of Scrambled Eggs with Spinach and Feta for a protein-packed start to your day.

Snack: Grab a handful of Mixed Nuts for a convenient and satisfying mid-morning snack to keep your energy levels up.

Lunch: Dive into the refreshing flavors of a Chicken and Avocado Wrap, filled with lean protein and healthy fats to keep you satisfied.

Snack: Satisfy your sweet tooth with a serving of Apple Slices with Almond Butter, offering a deliciously crunchy and satisfying snack.

Dinner: Indulge in the savory goodness of Grilled Chicken with Roasted Vegetables, offering a satisfying blend of protein and fiber to keep you full and satisfied.

Dessert: Treat yourself to a creamy and indulgent serving of Greek Yogurt with Honey and Walnuts, offering a satisfyingly sweet and crunchy dessert option.

Day 16

Breakfast: Start your day with the refreshing flavors of a Berry Smoothie Bowl, topped with granola and shredded coconut for added texture and sweetness.

Snack: Keep your energy levels up with a serving of Cottage Cheese with Pineapple, offering a satisfying blend of protein and natural sweetness.

Lunch: Dive into the hearty goodness of Lentil Soup with Mixed Vegetables, offering a satisfying blend of protein and fiber to keep you full and satisfied.

Snack: Enjoy the crunchy goodness of Carrot Sticks with Hummus, offering a nutritious and flavorful snack to keep you fueled throughout the day.

Dinner: Indulge in the savory flavors of Baked Cod with Quinoa Pilaf, offering a deliciously satisfying meal that's perfect for any time of day.

Dessert: Treat yourself to a sweet and satisfying serving of Dark Chocolate Bark with Almonds and Sea Salt, offering a deliciously indulgent dessert option.

Day 17

Breakfast: Wake up to the delightful flavors of Banana Oatmeal Pancakes, topped with fresh fruit and a drizzle of maple syrup for a sweet and satisfying start to your day.

Snack: Keep your energy levels up with a serving of Greek Yogurt with Berries and Granola, offering a satisfying blend of protein, fiber, and complex carbohydrates.

Lunch: Dive into the refreshing flavors of a Caprese Salad with Balsamic Glaze, offering a light and flavorful meal that's perfect for a midday pick-me-up.

Snack: Enjoy the creamy goodness of Avocado Toast with Cherry Tomatoes, offering a satisfying blend of healthy fats and fiber to keep you full and satisfied.

Dinner: Indulge in the savory flavors of Spaghetti Squash with Turkey Meatballs and Marinara Sauce, offering a satisfyingly hearty meal that's perfect for any time of day.

Dessert: Treat yourself to a sweet and satisfying serving of Coconut Chia Pudding with Fresh Mango, offering a deliciously tropical dessert option.

Day 18

Breakfast: Start your day with the savory flavors of a Veggie Egg Scramble, filled with mushrooms, bell peppers, onions, and spinach for a nutritious and satisfying meal.

Snack: Keep your energy levels up with a serving of Trail Mix with Dried Fruit and Nuts, offering a satisfying blend of protein, fiber, and natural sweetness.

Lunch: Dive into the hearty goodness of a Turkey and Avocado Wrap with Whole Grain Bread, offering a satisfying blend of lean protein, healthy fats, and complex carbohydrates.

Snack: Enjoy the crunchy goodness of Bell Pepper Strips with Guacamole, offering a satisfyingly savory and nutritious snack option.

Dinner: Indulge in the savory flavors of a Beef Stir-Fry with Broccoli and Brown Rice, offering a deliciously satisfying meal that's perfect for any time of day.

Dessert: Treat yourself to a sweet and satisfying serving of Frozen Yogurt Bark with Berries and Granola, offering a deliciously refreshing dessert option.

Day 19

Breakfast: Wake up to the delightful flavors of Peanut Butter and Banana Overnight Oats, offering a satisfyingly creamy and indulgent breakfast option.

Snack: Keep your energy levels up with a serving of Mixed Berry Smoothie, offering a deliciously refreshing and nutritious snack option.

Lunch: Dive into the refreshing flavors of a Greek Salad with Grilled Chicken, offering a light and flavorful meal that's perfect for a midday pick-me-up.

Snack: Enjoy the creamy goodness of Cottage Cheese with Tomato Slices and Basil, offering a satisfyingly savory and nutritious snack option.

Dinner: Indulge in the savory flavors of Baked Salmon with Asparagus and Quinoa, offering a deliciously satisfying meal that's perfect for any time of day.

Dessert: Treat yourself to a sweet and satisfying serving of Strawberry Banana Nice Cream, offering a deliciously refreshing and guilt-free dessert option.

Day 20

Breakfast: Start your day with the hearty flavors of a Breakfast Burrito with Scrambled Eggs, Black Beans, and Salsa, offering a satisfyingly savory and nutritious meal.

Snack: Keep your energy levels up with a serving of Apple Slices with Almond Butter and Cinnamon, offering a deliciously sweet and satisfying snack option.

Lunch: Dive into the refreshing flavors of a Quinoa Salad with Chickpeas, Cucumber, and Feta, offering a light and flavorful meal that's perfect for a midday pick-me-up.

Snack: Enjoy the crunchy goodness of Celery Sticks with Peanut Butter and Raisins, offering a satisfyingly savory and nutritious snack option.

Dinner: Indulge in the savory flavors of Grilled Chicken Caesar Salad with Whole Grain Croutons, offering a deliciously satisfying meal that's perfect for any time of day.

Dessert: Treat yourself to a sweet and satisfying serving of Dark Chocolate Covered Strawberries, offering a deliciously indulgent and guilt-free dessert option.

Day 21

Breakfast: Start your day with a nutritious serving of Overnight Chia Seed Pudding with Mixed Berries, offering a satisfying blend of fiber and antioxidants to fuel your morning.

Snack: Keep your energy levels up with a handful of Cashews and Dried Apricots, providing a satisfying mix of healthy fats and natural sweetness.

Lunch: Dive into the refreshing flavors of a Spinach and Strawberry Salad with Grilled Chicken, drizzled with balsamic vinaigrette for a light and satisfying meal.

Snack: Enjoy the crunchy goodness of Snap Pea Crisps, offering a flavorful and nutritious snack to keep you energized throughout the day.

Dinner: Indulge in the savory goodness of Baked Halibut with Lemon and Herbs, served with a side of roasted Brussels sprouts for a delicious and nutritious dinner.

Dessert: Treat yourself to a sweet and satisfying serving of Greek Yogurt with Honey and Sliced Almonds, offering a creamy and indulgent dessert option.

Day 22

Breakfast: Wake up to the delicious flavors of Banana Almond Butter Toast, topped with sliced bananas and a sprinkle of cinnamon for a comforting and nutritious breakfast.

Snack: Keep your energy levels up with a serving of Whole Grain Crackers with Goat Cheese and Cherry Tomatoes, offering a satisfying blend of protein and fiber.

Lunch: Dive into the hearty goodness of Lentil Salad with Roasted Vegetables, offering a satisfying mix of protein, fiber, and complex carbohydrates to keep you full and satisfied.

Snack: Enjoy the refreshing flavors of Watermelon Cubes with Feta and Mint, offering a light and hydrating snack option that's perfect for hot summer days.

Dinner: Indulge in the savory flavors of Turkey Meatballs with Zucchini Noodles, served with marinara sauce and freshly grated Parmesan cheese for a satisfying and nutritious meal.

Dessert: Treat yourself to a sweet and satisfying serving of Baked Apple with Cinnamon and Greek Yogurt, offering a warm and comforting dessert option.

Day 23

Breakfast: Start your day with a refreshing and energizing Green Smoothie, packed with spinach, kale, banana, and pineapple for a nutritious and delicious morning boost.

Snack: Keep your energy levels up with a serving of Sliced Bell Peppers with Hummus, offering a satisfying blend of crunchy vegetables and creamy dip.

Lunch: Dive into the satisfying flavors of a Mediterranean Chickpea Salad, tossed with cucumbers, tomatoes, red onion, olives, and feta cheese in a lemon herb dressing.

Snack: Enjoy the sweet and tangy flavors of Greek Yogurt with Mango and Granola, offering a satisfyingly creamy and crunchy snack option.

Dinner: Indulge in the savory goodness of Baked Cod with Herbed Quinoa Pilaf, served with a side of steamed broccoli for a nutritious and delicious dinner.

Dessert: Treat yourself to a sweet and satisfying serving of Mixed Berry Parfait with Vanilla Yogurt and Almond Granola, offering a refreshing and indulgent dessert option.

Day 24

Breakfast: Wake up to the comforting flavors of Apple Cinnamon Baked Oatmeal, served warm with a dollop of Greek yogurt for added creaminess.

Snack: Keep your energy levels up with a serving of Trail Mix with Dark Chocolate Chips, offering a satisfying blend of nuts, seeds, and dried fruit for a tasty and nutritious snack.

Lunch: Dive into the hearty goodness of a Turkey and Avocado Wrap with Whole Grain Tortilla, filled with sliced turkey breast, avocado, lettuce, tomato, and mustard for a satisfying and flavorful meal.

Snack: Enjoy the refreshing flavors of Cucumber Slices with Tzatziki Sauce, offering a light and hydrating snack option that's perfect for warm summer days.

Dinner: Indulge in the savory flavors of Lemon Garlic Shrimp with Quinoa and Steamed Asparagus, offering a light and nutritious meal that's bursting with flavor.

Dessert: Treat yourself to a sweet and satisfying serving of Chocolate Covered Strawberries, offering a deliciously indulgent and guilt-free dessert option.

Day 25

Breakfast: Start your day with a hearty and nutritious serving of Breakfast Burrito Bowl, made with scrambled eggs, black beans, diced avocado, salsa, and shredded cheese for a satisfying and flavorful meal.

Snack: Keep your energy levels up with a serving of Greek Yogurt with Berries and Almond Butter, offering a satisfying blend of protein, fiber, and healthy fats.

Lunch: Dive into the refreshing flavors of a Caprese Salad with Balsamic Glaze, made with fresh mozzarella cheese, ripe tomatoes, fresh basil leaves, and a drizzle of balsamic glaze for a light and flavorful meal.

Snack: Enjoy the crunchy goodness of Carrot Sticks with Ranch Dip, offering a satisfyingly crunchy and flavorful snack option that's perfect for any time of day.

Dinner: Indulge in the savory flavors of Baked Chicken with Roasted Sweet Potatoes and Brussels Sprouts, offering a hearty and nutritious meal that's perfect for chilly evenings.

Dessert: Treat yourself to a sweet and satisfying serving of Mixed Berry Crisp with Vanilla Greek Yogurt, offering a deliciously fruity and comforting dessert option.

Day 26

Breakfast: Wake up to the delicious flavors of Peanut Butter Banana Overnight Oats, made with rolled oats, almond milk, peanut butter, sliced banana, and a sprinkle of cinnamon for a nutritious and satisfying breakfast option.

Snack: Keep your energy levels up with a serving of Apple Slices with Almond Butter and Honey, offering a satisfying blend of sweet and savory flavors.

Lunch: Dive into the hearty goodness of Lentil Soup with Crusty Whole Grain Bread, offering a satisfying blend of protein, fiber, and complex carbohydrates to keep you full and satisfied.

Snack: Enjoy the refreshing flavors of Watermelon Cubes with Feta and Mint, offering a light and hydrating snack option that's perfect for warm summer days.

Dinner: Indulge in the savory flavors of Turkey Stuffed Bell Peppers with Quinoa and Black Beans, offering a deliciously satisfying meal that's packed with protein and fiber.

Dessert: Treat yourself to a sweet and satisfying serving of Banana "Nice" Cream with Dark Chocolate Chips and Almond Butter, offering a guilt-free and indulgent dessert option.

Day 27

Breakfast: Start your day with a refreshing and energizing Green Smoothie Bowl, made with spinach, kale, banana, pineapple, and almond milk, topped with granola, sliced banana, and a drizzle of honey for added sweetness.

Snack: Keep your energy levels up with a serving of Mixed Nuts and Dried Fruit, offering a satisfying blend of protein, healthy fats, and natural sweetness.

Lunch: Dive into the satisfying flavors of a Mediterranean Chickpea Salad Wrap, filled with chickpeas, cucumber, tomato, red onion, feta cheese, and a drizzle of tahini sauce for a flavorful and nutritious meal.

Snack: Enjoy the crunchy goodness of Celery Sticks with Peanut Butter and Raisins, offering a satisfyingly sweet and savory snack option.

Dinner: Indulge in the savory flavors of Grilled Salmon with Roasted Vegetables and Quinoa, offering a deliciously satisfying meal that's packed with protein, fiber, and essential nutrients.

Dessert: Treat yourself to a sweet and satisfying serving of Greek Yogurt with Honey and Sliced Almonds, offering a creamy and indulgent dessert option.

Day 28

Breakfast: Wake up to the comforting flavors of Banana Walnut Baked Oatmeal Cups, made with ripe bananas, chopped walnuts, rolled oats, almond milk, and a touch of maple syrup for a deliciously satisfying breakfast option.

Snack: Keep your energy levels up with a serving of Whole Grain Crackers with Goat Cheese and Cherry

Tomatoes, offering a satisfying blend of protein, fiber, and complex carbohydrates.

Lunch: Dive into the refreshing flavors of a Greek Salad with Grilled Chicken, made with crisp lettuce, juicy tomatoes, cucumber, red onion, kalamata olives, feta cheese, and a tangy Greek dressing for a light and satisfying meal.

Snack: Enjoy the sweet and tangy flavors of Greek Yogurt with Mango and Granola, offering a satisfyingly creamy and crunchy snack option.

Dinner: Indulge in the savory flavors of Baked Cod with Herbed Quinoa Pilaf, served with a side of steamed broccoli for a deliciously satisfying meal that's packed with protein and fiber.

Dessert: Treat yourself to a sweet and satisfying serving of Mixed Berry Parfait with Vanilla Yogurt and Almond Granola, offering a refreshing and indulgent dessert option.

Day 29

Breakfast: Start your day with a nutritious and delicious serving of Blueberry Almond Butter Smoothie, made with frozen blueberries, almond butter, Greek yogurt, almond milk, and a touch of honey for a satisfying and energizing breakfast option.

Snack: Keep your energy levels up with a serving of Trail Mix with Dark Chocolate Chips, offering a satisfying blend of nuts, seeds, and dried fruit for a tasty and nutritious snack.

Lunch: Dive into the hearty goodness of a Turkey and Avocado Wrap with Whole Grain Tortilla, filled with sliced turkey breast, avocado, lettuce, tomato, and mustard for a satisfying and flavorful meal.

Snack: Enjoy the refreshing flavors of Cucumber Slices with Tzatziki Sauce, offering a light and hydrating snack option that's perfect for warm summer days.

Dinner: Indulge in the savory flavors of Lemon Garlic Shrimp with Quinoa and Steamed Asparagus, offering a light and nutritious meal that's bursting with flavor.

Dessert: Treat yourself to a sweet and satisfying serving of Chocolate Covered Strawberries, offering a deliciously indulgent and guilt-free dessert option.

Day 30

Breakfast: Wake up to the comforting flavors of Apple Cinnamon Baked Oatmeal, served warm with a dollop of Greek yogurt for added creaminess.

Snack: Keep your energy levels up with a serving of Trail Mix with Dark Chocolate Chips, offering a satisfying blend of nuts, seeds, and dried fruit for a tasty and nutritious snack.

Lunch: Dive into the refreshing flavors of a Caprese Salad with Balsamic Glaze, made with fresh mozzarella cheese, ripe tomatoes, fresh basil leaves, and a drizzle of balsamic glaze for a light and flavorful meal.

Snack: Enjoy the crunchy goodness of Carrot Sticks with Ranch Dip, offering a satisfyingly crunchy and flavorful snack option that's perfect for any time of day.

Dinner: Indulge in the savory flavors of Baked Chicken with Roasted Sweet Potatoes and Brussels Sprouts, offering a hearty and nutritious meal that's perfect for chilly evenings.

Dessert: Treat yourself to a sweet and satisfying serving of Mixed Berry Crisp with Vanilla Greek Yogurt, offering a deliciously fruity and comforting dessert option.

This 30-day meal plan offers a diverse array of nutrient-dense, low glycemic recipes designed to nourish the body and support overall health and wellness. By incorporating a variety of whole foods, lean proteins, healthy fats, and complex carbohydrates, this meal plan provides balanced nutrition while helping to stabilize blood sugar levels and promote long-term satiety.

Throughout the plan, there's an emphasis on flavorful and satisfying meals that are both enjoyable to eat and beneficial for health. From hearty breakfast options to light and refreshing lunches, and comforting dinners, each day offers a delicious and nutritious lineup of meals and snacks.

Conclusion

Embracing a low glycemic diet isn't just about managing blood sugar levels; it's about embracing a lifestyle that prioritizes health and well-being. Throughout this book, we've explored the principles of low glycemic eating and discovered how it can positively impact our energy levels, weight management, and overall health.

By incorporating the tips and recipes provided in this book, you have the opportunity to transform your relationship with food and nourish your body with delicious, nutrient-dense meals. Whether you're enjoying a hearty breakfast, a satisfying lunch, or a flavorful dinner, each recipe has been carefully crafted to support your health goals while tantalizing your taste buds.

But beyond the recipes, adopting a low glycemic lifestyle opens the door to a world of possibilities. It's about making mindful choices, listening to your body, and finding joy in nourishing yourself with wholesome foods. It's about recognizing that every meal is an opportunity to fuel your body, support your well-being, and live your best life.

As you continue on your journey, remember that consistency is key. Embrace the process, celebrate your successes, and don't be afraid to experiment with new flavors and ingredients. And above all, be kind to yourself. Health is a journey, not a destination, and every step you take towards nourishing your body is a step in the right direction.

So here's to you, and here's to the delicious, nutritious meals that await. May your plates be full, your hearts be light, and your health be vibrant for years to come. Cheers to a lifetime of low glycemic living and all the joy it brings.

By following this meal plan, individuals can experience a wide range of health benefits, including improved energy levels, better blood sugar control, enhanced weight management, and overall well-being. Additionally, the inclusion of snacks and desserts ensures that cravings are satisfied without compromising on nutritional quality.

Ultimately, this meal plan serves as a valuable resource for individuals looking to adopt a low glycemic eating approach while enjoying delicious and satisfying meals. With careful planning and preparation, it's possible to maintain a healthy and balanced diet that supports optimal health and vitality for the long term.

Daily Meal Remark

Day	Recipes	Remark